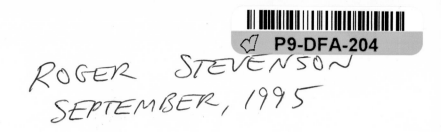

ROGER STEVENSON
SEPTEMBER, 1995

Gender, Health, and Longevity

Marcia G. Ory, Ph.D., M.P.H., is Chief, Social Science Research on Aging, Behavioral and Social Research Program, National Institute on Aging, National Institutes of Health, Bethesda, Maryland. She holds a doctorate from Purdue University and a Masters of Public Health from The Johns Hopkins University. Dr. Ory is very active in professional organizations and serves on several national task forces and advisory boards dealing with aging and health issues. Her main areas of interest include aging and health care, health and behavior research, and gender differences in health and longevity. She has published widely on these topics.

Huber R. Warner, Ph.D., is Deputy Associate Director of the Biomedical Research and Clinical Medicine Program and Chief of the Molecular and Cell Biology Branch in the National Institute on Aging where he has been since 1984. From 1964 through 1984 he was on the faculty of the Department of Biochemistry at the University of Minnesota, where his research focused on the metabolism of nucleic acids and replication of viruses.

Jacquelyn Scarville, M.A., is a Research Sociologist in the Manpower Personnel Research Laboratory, Army Research Institute, and a doctoral candidate in sociology at the University of Maryland, College Park. During 1989 she worked with the National Institute on Aging on projects related to gender and aging. She has presented papers on military spouse employment and is currently working on a dissertation investigating the determinants of job autonomy.

Gender, Health, and Longevity

Multidisciplinary Perspectives

Marcia G. Ory
Huber R. Warner

Editors

With the assistance of Jacquelyn Scarville

Foreword by
Matilda White Riley

Springer Publishing Company
New York

Springer Publishing Company, Inc.
536 Broadway
New York, NY 10012

90 91 92 93 94 / 5 4 3 2 1

Library of Congress Cataloging-in-Publication Data

Gender, health, and longevity : multidisciplinary perspectives /
     edited by Marcia G. Ory, Huber R. Warner with the assistance of
     Jacquelyn Scarville ; foreword by Matilda White Riley.
          p.   cm.
     Includes bibliographical references.
     ISBN 0–8261–7140–0
     1. Longevity—Sex differences.   2. Health—Sex differences.
I. Ory, Marcia G.   II. Warner, Huber R.
QP85.G38   90-35541
1990   616.6'8—dc20   CIP

Printed in the United States of America

Contents

Foreword: The Gender Paradox

This book revisits a familiar but still puzzling paradox: in the United States today, on the average, at every age women report more illness and health care utilization than men, yet life expectancy is consistently higher for women than for men. Many questions have been raised, but few satisfactory answers have been given. What are the sources of such striking differences between the sexes? What accounts for the reversal between the sexes in patterns of health and longevity? What is the significance of this fact that women have higher levels of morbidity, but live longer? What are the implications for research? For public policy? For professional practice?

These remain among the most serious and most perplexing questions of our time. The few answers now being offered, and the actions now being taken on the basis of these answers, will have untold consequences for the future. These consequences will ramify throughout all sectors of society. They will touch the lives of every individual. Thus it is not too soon to reformulate the pertinent questions more precisely, to seek answers through more systematic and powerful research designs, and to provide a more detailed knowledge base for implementation and intervention.

SOURCES OF DIFFERENCE

The current longevity and health differences between men and women have been developing for many decades. They arise from diverse and complex changes in the society as a whole, changes that have been swirling around us so rapidly that they often go unnoticed. Over two-thirds of the increases in longevity that have occurred throughout all history have taken place during our own century. These increases have had unequal impact on the two sexes. In this country in 1900, life expectancy at birth was almost equal—about 48 years for men and 51 for women. Today the gender gap in longevity has widened to a 7-year difference—between 71 for men and 78 for women.[1] This widening gap has been associated with other century-long societal changes: drastic reductions in childbearing; improvements in standard of living and public health; advances in science and medicine; the shift from acute to chronic diseases; dramatic increases in female entry into the labor force; and other secular changes that are at once social, behavioral, and biomedical.

Such trends are still continuing, and they have proven to be too transitory and too massive in scope to be fully encompassed in the literatures of science. Yet, among scholars in discrete fields, many separate sources of sex differences have long been recognized. Let me rehearse a few of the things we thought we already knew about gender differences in longevity and in health back in the 1960s (when I was involved in preparation of an inventory of social science findings on aging and society [Riley, Foner, Moore, Hess, & Roth, 1968]).

With regard to longevity, many indications of genetic influences had already been well established. Females were found to outlive males even in fetal life (where more male than female stillbirths were noted), and also in most other mammalian animal species. At the same time, many other indications pointed to sociocultural influences on longevity, as the historical changes and their societal correlates attest.

The combined effects of nature and nurture were also clearly apparent with regard to gender differences in health and illness, as these too were described in that inventory of more than two decades ago. We knew then how many of the biological factors were modulated or even caused by changing sociocultural conditions. We knew that older men and women suffer from different types of morbidity—men from comparatively more lethal diseases, such as heart disease; women from comparatively more disabling conditions, such as diabetes, rheumatoid arthritis, and osteoporosis. We knew in the 1960s that the increased smoking among incoming cohorts of young women would tend to result by the 1980s in increased death rates from cancer—just as we can now anticipate future tendencies toward decline in cancer death rates for both women and men as current cohorts of young adults are now reducing the rates of smoking.

In short, some of the central sources of gender differences had already been identified two decades ago. In the succeeding years, countless further research findings have been reported. For example, studies have examined how the expression of hormonal differences between the sexes is modulated by the stressful conditions associated with gender roles at work or in the family, or by the ability of individuals to cope with such stresses. Research has examined the health consequences of the differing life-styles and roles of men and women that involve smoking, exercise, diet, violence, and other risk factors. Still other findings show how men and women perceive and act on symptoms differently; how older women engage in more preventive care than do older men; how women tend to use more physician visits, while men use more hospital care.

RESEARCH APPROACHES

As knowledge of gender differences has been accumulating, methods and conceptual frameworks for understanding these differences—their sources, consequences, and the mechanisms involved—have been developing. The emerging approaches, some of which are illustrated in this book, include:

- The use of historical research as a laboratory for testing hypotheses about gender differences. History, although we rarely think of it in laboratory terms, is fast coming to be recognized, like cross-cultural comparison, as a powerful research tool.
- The investigation of genetic and neuroscientific mechanisms, as genetic predispositions come to be understood as interacting with endocrine, immunological, neural, and other physiological systems to affect health and longevity.
- The revolution in social science methodology, which informs longitudinal and cohort approaches to research on health and longevity.
- The long-neglected development of studies focused on women, to counterbalance those focused exclusively on men. Studies of women are in turn prompting deeper analyses of the factors in health and longevity among men, and of the gender differences in these factors.

- The gradual recognition of the need for specification, as research goes beyond global explanations to specify how, and under what conditions, specific sex and gender characteristics influence health and longevity. For example, many earlier studies simply generalized about the presumed negative impact on men of retirement, and on women of widowhood. However, these generalizations broke down as the data made clear that there are no generally negative outcomes of these transitions. Instead, there are wide variations among individuals of both sexes, and among the surrounding circumstances. The outcome is now seen to depend in large part on specific intervening processes—such as coping style, or affective ties toward the particular spouse or the particular job that has been lost.

- Perhaps most important of all the scientific developments is recognition of the need for multidisciplinary communication. Further advance is awaiting fuller integration of the developments that have been occurring in the separate scientific disciplines. Even the basic terms are discipline-specific: "sex," to convey the biological meaning; "gender," to emphasize the sociocultural. Yet, it is the linkages among biological, behavioral, social, and cultural processes that are most markedly affecting health and longevity in both males and females. Understanding of these linkages requires multidisciplinary perspectives.

NEED FOR THIS BOOK

Multidisciplinary communication is not easy to come by, however. To achieve it is one of the major goals of this book. Indeed, even two decades ago it would have been impossible to assemble the multidisciplinary contributions represented here.

Conversations among these contributors began in 1987 at a symposium held at the annual meetings of the American Association for the Advancement of Science in Chicago, Illinois. That symposium was aptly titled "Gender, Health, and Longevity: Multidisciplinary Perspectives." Thoughtful papers and provocative discussions went far toward defining the central questions; but they were only a small beginning toward answering the questions.

Later in 1987 further and more extensive efforts toward answers were made at a conference held by the National Institute on Aging on "Gender and Longevity" in Bethesda, Maryland. A number of the papers from that conference, supplemented by others, were subsequently revised and reviewed by outside experts and they are published here.

SIGNIFICANCE OF THE BOOK

The chapters in this volume provide much information and many ideas from several disciplines about the still unexplained paradox before us: that, on the average and under today's conditions, women have higher levels of illness and disability than men, yet they live longer. As these chapters itemize the gender differences, and as they seek to account for them, they point to implications that far transcend the immediate gender issue of health and longevity. These implications go to the heart of many larger and longer-range issues that will predictably confront science, policy, and professional practice in many domains and for many years to come.

The increase in longevity will alone have untold consequences. Longevity allows recent cohorts of young people to stay in school longer than their predecessors did, foreshadowing increases in the level of education of old people of the future. Longevity prolongs retirement. It postpones many of the diseases of old age. It extends family relationships—as husbands and wives now typically survive together for four, even five, decades or more. All such consequences of longevity impinge on men and women in different ways, affecting both society and individual lives.

Because women are living longer than men, the society as a whole is becoming a society of older women. Already there are three older women for every two older men. Most older men are married and live in a family setting, whereas most older women are widowed. Among those 75 and over, more than half of the women are living alone, in contrast to less than one-fifth of the men (U.S. Senate Special Committee on Aging, 1988).[2] For these cohorts of women, for whom marriage and keeping house was the major activity, many have lost their traditional places in society.

Because life experiences of men and women differ, their extended lives will raise many questions about the cohorts of men and women who will be old in the future. How, for example, will husbands and wives adapt to retirement? Will the many wives currently in the labor force, who are typically younger than their husbands, continue to work after their husbands have retired? Such a change would produce a new stage in the family cycle, a stage of "husband retirement," requiring entirely new patterns of living for the individuals involved. Or, to take another example, how will women's role as family caregiver be affected, if long-lived wives are often preoccupied with the care of a frail husband to the point where the wives can no longer care even for themselves?

Perhaps the most critical of all the questions concerns the health of those whose lives are prolonged. The arguments over "compression of morbidity" within the last years of life still persist (cf., Fries, Green, Levine, 1989)[3]: but it is clear that modern medicine allows many individuals to be kept alive through long years of disability and illness, while many other individuals—the majority—retain into old age their vigor and ability to function (cf., Riley & Bond, 1983).[4] The gender issue concerns the balance between disability and functioning among very old women as compared with very old men. Kenneth Manton reports in this volume that, among that minority of the very old who are similarly disabled, it is the women who survive longer than the men. Will these disabled older women demonstrate the resilience and capacity to cope that so far have characterized older women in general? Will the future bring improved health for both sexes? Is it possible that reduced risks in the life-styles of men will extend their longevity to that of women, as in the query by Constance Nathanson in this volume?

Such are the issues, often still perplexing, that are presented in the chapters of this book. Some are inscrutable. Most, however, provide fertile ground, not only for further research, but also for viable and feasible interventions. Interventions are essential for enhancing health and the quality of life for both sexes. And research is essential for guiding interventions, pending full resolution of the paradox that this volume sets out in such tantalizing detail.

MATILDA WHITE RILEY
National Institute on Aging

NOTES

1. Estimates of longevity vary somewhat, depending on methods of calculation; and of course, they are subject to change over time.

2. These data refer to 1986 in the United States, but all such demographic data are subject to the rapid changes currently underway.

3. Despite repeated criticisms, James Fries still contends that the upper boundary of life expectancy has already been reached.

4. The notion that the onset of disability could be postponed does not necessarily imply, as Fries argues, that the outer boundary of life expectancy has already been reached.

REFERENCES

Fries, J. L., Green, L. R., & Levine, S. (March 4, 1989). Health promotion and the compression of morbidity. *Lancet,* 482.

Riley, M. W., & Bond, K. (1983). Beyond ageism: Postponing the onset of disability. In M. W. Riley, B. B. Hess, & K. Bond (Eds.), *Aging and society* (pp. 243–252). Hillsdale, NJ: Erlbaum.

Riley, M. W., Foner, A., Moore, M. E., Hess, B., & Roth, B. K. (1968). *Aging and society: I. An inventory of research findings.* New York: Russell Sage Foundation.

U.S. Senate Special Committee on Aging. (1987–1988). *Aging America: Trends and projections* (p. 4). Washington, DC: U.S. Government Printing Office.

Acknowledgments

The publication of such a multidisciplinary volume as this has presented particular challenges to the editors and we acknowledge the assistance of many of our colleagues. We especially acknowledge the interest and encouragement of T. Franklin Williams, Matilda White Riley, Edward L. Schneider, and Richard L. Sprott during the conceptual phases of this project. This encouragement led first to a symposium organized by Matilda White Riley titled "Gender, Health and Longevity: Multidisciplinary Perspectives" which was held at the annual meeting of the American Association for the Advancement of Sciences in February, 1987. This was followed by a major symposium organized by National Institute on Aging (NIA) staff on "Gender and longevity: Why do women live longer than men?" which was held in Bethesda, Maryland in September, 1987. We are especially grateful to Dr. David W. E. Smith for his help in organizing this symposium while on sabbatical at NIA. The presentations at these two symposia form the basis for many of the chapters included here. Jacquelyn Scarville deserves special recognition for her assistance throughout all phases of the editing process. We are also indebted to Alan R. Price, Matilda White Riley, Diego Segre, Diane Zablotsky, and Karin Mack for reading and assisting with the editing of these manuscripts. Finally, we thank Diane Foltin, Hollie Keylor, Claudette Grubelich and Michelle Blanco whose work behind the scenes was crucial to the success of the symposium and the publication of this volume.

Contributors

Donald J. Brambilla, Ph.D., has a background in biostatistics and biology. He is currently a Senior Research Scientist at the New England Research Institute, Watertown, Massachusetts. Most recently he has worked as the statistician on a large, longitudinal study of the health of middle-aged women. His current research interests include survey methods, the validity of survey data, and the analysis of longitudinal data. His most recent publications include papers on factors affecting age at menopause, the validity of self-reports of cancer incidence, and a comparison of responses to telephone and face-to-face interviews in a longitudinal study.

Barbara A. Cohn, Ph.D., is a Senior Research Scientist with the California Public Health Foundation in Berkeley, California. She holds a doctoral degree in Epidemiology and masters degree in City and Regional Planning, and Public Health Planning and Administration from the University of California, Berkeley and is interested in the development and application of new methodologic approaches to epidemiologic questions and health policy. Her research has included a new use of twin data to study cardiovascular disease risk in women, gender differences in health and mortality, and the time paths of these differences over the lifespan, and the infant health consequences of adolescent pregnancy.

Matthew B. Ferdock, B.S., has a background in Applied Psychology and statistics; he currently works as a Research Associate with the

New England Research Institute. His professional interests have included manuscripts and presentations on statistics, social support, drug use, and reliability of survey data.

Stanley M. Gartler, Ph.D., is Professor of Medicine and Genetics at the University of Washington, where he has taught since 1957. He is past president of the American Society for Human Genetics. Dr. Gartler has worked on mammalian X-chromosome inactivation for the past twenty-five years and is responsible for the ideas and direction of work on the molecular cytology of X-chromosomes and methylation analysis of several specific loci.

William R. Hazzard, M.D., is Professor and Chairman of the Department of Internal Medicine at the Bowman Gray School of Medicine of Wake Forest University. Dr. Hazzard's career has focused on the relationship between sex steroids and lipoprotein transport and incidence of coronary disease in humans. As his career turned more toward gerontology in the 1970s, he became particularly interested in the role of estrogens and androgens in the sex differential in longevity. His professional commitment to developing and retaining gerontology and geriatric medicine within the mainstream of the American academic medical establishment places him in a unique position among American geriatricians.

Howard R. Kelman, Ph.D., a medical sociologist, is Director of the Division of Health Services Organization and Policy and is a Professor in the Department of Epidemiology and Social Medicine of Montefiore Medical Center and Albert Einstein College of Medicine. Over the course of his career in research and teaching, he has conducted a variety of sociomedical studies here and abroad with an emphasis on long-term and chronic illness, rehabilitation and disability, health service use and health care evaluation. These studies and his extensive publications have included experimental assessments of nursing home patients, studies of disabled and chronically ill children and adults, merchant seamen, and more recently, longitudinal studies of aging, health, and health care.

Kenneth G. Manton, Ph.D., is Research Professor of Demographic Studies at Duke University and Medical Research Professor at Duke University Medical Center's Department of Community and Family Medicine. Dr. Manton is also a Senior Fellow of the Duke University Medical Center's Center for the Study of Aging and Human Development and Research Director of the Duke University Center for

Demographic Studies. In 1986 he was named head of the World Health Organization Collaborating Center for Research and Training in the Methods of Assessing Risk and Forecasting Health Status Trends as Related to Multiple Disease Outcomes, based at the Center for Demographic Studies. His current research interests include forecasting morbidity, disability, and mortality among the nation's elderly, reimbursement maintenance of quality of care for both acute and long-term care services consumed by the elderly, mathematical modeling at advanced ages, and differentials in those processes by sex and race and cross-nationality. He has published extensively in these areas, including a book with Eric Stallard, *Chronic Disease Modelling: Measurement and Evaluation of the Risk of Chronic Disease Processes.*

John B. McKinlay, Ph.D., is Vice-President and Director of the New England Research Institute, a private research organization specializing in epidemiology, gerontology, health services research, and social policy. He is also Professor of Sociology and Research Professor of Medicine at Boston University, and holds appointments at the Beth Israel and Massachusetts General Hospitals (Harvard Medical School). He has published numerous books and professional papers, and is a consultant to national governments, state agencies, and international organizations on matters of health and social policy issues. In 1987 he received a prestigious MERIT Award from the National Institutes of Health.

Sonja M. McKinlay, Ph.D., is a Statistician/Epidemiologist who is President and Co-Owner of New England Research Institute, Watertown, Massachusetts and Associate Professor of Community Health at Brown University, Rhode Island. Her publications encompass statistical methodology as well as cardiovascular and reproductive epidemiology. Most recently she has authored papers on aspects of menopause arising from a large longitudinal study of the health of middle-aged women, for which she is the principal investigator.

Constance A. Nathanson, Ph.D., is a Professor in the Department of Population Dynamics at the Johns Hopkins University School of Hygiene and Public Health and Director of the Hopkins Population Center. She has published extensively on sociological dimensions of women's reproductive health and on sex differences in health and mortality. She is currently completing a book on the social and historical context of adolescent pregnancy as a public problem and is engaged in research on the determinants of sexual and protective behavior among male and female sexually transmitted disease (STD) clinic clients.

James V. Neel, M.D., is Lee R. Dice Distinguished University Professor of Human Genetics, Emeritus, at the University of Michigan, where he was Chairman of its Department of Human Genetics for 25 years. He has authored numerous articles on human genetics, with a particular current interest in the genetic structure of unacculturated Amerindian tribes and in human mutation rates, with special reference to the potential genetic impact of the atomic bombs.

Matilda White Riley, D.Sc., is Associate Director of Behavioral and Social Research, National Institute on Aging, National Institutes of Health, and Professor Emerita of Sociology at Rutgers University and Bowdoin College. She is a member of the American Academy of Arts and Sciences and the Institute of Medicine (National Academy of Sciences). She has received an honorary L.H.D. and the Common Wealth Award in Sociology. Her publications include *Sociological Research, Sociological Studies in Scale Analysis, Aging and Society, Aging from Birth to Death, Social Change and the Life Course,* and numerous articles on mass communication, socialization, intergenerational relationships, and research methods.

David W. E. Smith, M.D., is a Professor of Pathology and Associate Director of the Center on Aging of Northwestern University Medical School. Having spent many years doing research on transfer RNA and details of its function in protein synthesis, he has recently turned his attention to aging and longevity. During a year-long sabbatical at the National Institute on Aging, he organized the Conference on Gender and Longevity: Why Do Women Live Longer Than Men? He has continued to publish on this question, particularly its genetic aspects, and he is currently doing research on aging in careers and on some considerations of life styles of elderly people.

Cynthia Thomas, Ph.D., has a doctorate in political science and is an Assistant Professor and Senior Research Associate in the Department of Epidemiology and Social Medicine at Montefiore Medical Center and Albert Einstein College of Medicine. Her research on public policy issues has been in the area of housing, health, and aging. She has conducted research on a broad range of topics related to survey research methodology, including most recently the development of indexes to measure hunger and issues related to the collection and analysis of longitudinal data.

Randi Triant, M.A., has a public affairs background with a strong emphasis on labor/management relations. Her current research interest focuses on differences in health care utilization and health symptomatology for unemployed and employed women.

Lois M. Verbrugge, Ph.D., is Full Research Scientist at the Institute of Gerontology, The University of Michigan. Her current research is on the leading chronic condition in mid- and late life—osteoarthritis—and its impact on physical and social functioning. Her other ongoing research interests include patterns of change in disability, trends and future prospects for Americans' health, and sex differentials in health and mortality. With a Special Emphasis Research Career Award from the National Institute on Aging, she has obtained biomedical training in the rheumatic diseases and is engaged in collaborative research with rheumatology colleagues.

Marc E. Weksler, M.D., is the Wright Professor of Geriatric Medicine at Cornell University Medical College and Director of the Division of Geriatrics and the New York Hospital-Cornell Medical Center. He also serves as chairman of the Immunology of Aging program of the World Health Organization and of the MKSAP Geriatric Committee of the American College of Physicians. His research interests center on the immunobiology of aging and the pathogenesis of the diseases of the elderly.

Deborah L. Wingard, Ph.D., is an Associate Professor of Epidemiology at the Medical School of the University of California in San Diego. She has published extensively on gender differences in morbidity, mortality, and lifestyle, using United States vital statistics data and data from two prospective population-based studies; the Alameda County Study and the Rancho Bernardo Study. Her work has focused on the joint effects of social, behavioral, and biological factors on gender differences in health.

Introduction: Gender, Health, and Aging: Not Just a Women's Issue

GENDER DIFFERENCES AS A MAJOR AGING ISSUE

The health and effective functioning of older persons is now a major concern to researchers, practitioners, and policymakers. Many important questions can be identified: Why do some people live longer than others? Does longer life translate into added years of quality life? What are the consequences of longer lives for families and society? Research is beginning to identify the role of biological, behavioral, and social factors in promoting health and preventing diseases and disabilities as people grow older (Binstock & Shanas, 1985; Birren & Schaie, 1985; Finch & Schneider, 1985; Ory & Bond, 1989; Riley, Hess, & Bond, 1983; U.S. Senate, 1988).

The simplistic view of aging as a "women's issue" comes from the observation that women predominate in old age. It belies the importance of examining well-documented gender differences in health and longevity that go beyond the mere counting of men and women at different ages. The reported differences between men and women can be viewed either in terms of women's relative advantages or men's relative disadvantages. In industrialized societies, women live longer than men, but report more illness and disability. The structure and variability of the gender gap, which may offer valuable clues to the reason for gender differences in longevity, are not well known.

PURPOSE OF THIS VOLUME

This volume documents differences in men's and women's health and longevity at different historical times and places, for individuals at different ages, for different illnesses and disabilities, and under different socioenvironmental conditions. Several explanations for gender differences are proposed, and the contributions of various genetic, biological, behavioral, and social influences are explored in depth. For example, we are beginning to recognize that there may be sex-related genetic codes and functions that influence relative longevity through their effects on hormonal and immunological systems.

Moreover, we are learning that some social roles, such as working outside the home, may not be detrimental to women, as previously assumed, and may even be beneficial. The consequences of gender differences in health and longevity are revealed in different patterns of health care utilization by men and women (e.g., men are more likely to be hospitalized; women to visit the doctor), and in different patterns of informal caregiving (e.g., women are consistently more likely than men to be both recipients and providers of informal care).

Going beyond the tendency of single-disciplinary studies to emphasize one factor or another, both biological constancies and social variabilities are recognized in this multidisciplinary volume. In fact most authors, whether from biological, behavioral, or social fields, conclude that discipline-specific variables are not sufficient to explain reported gender differences completely, and they call for additional interdisciplinary research. The underlying goal of this book is *not* to document the separate influences of biology and culture but rather to show the interactions of such influences in the real world. Special attention is given to the mechanisms by which social and behavioral variables, interacting with biological factors, influence gender differences, and how biological data and theories can be used to develop realistic population models of aging. Additionally, this volume goes beyond a simple comparison of gender differences in mortality to examine linkages among health, morbidity, disability, and mortality. The complexities in understanding gender differences in such health transitions become obvious. Under closer examination, the seemingly contradictory gender-related pattern for morbidity as opposed to mortality is reconciled. Sophisticated multivariate analyses are conducted to explore the circumstances under which reported gender differences in health and health care utilization will disappear. The persistence of gender differences when controlling for a wide range of social and behavioral factors gives credence to a fundamental genetic/biological difference between men and women. Similarly, the variability in the pattern of gender differences across various social categories attests to the importance of social explanations. We cannot neglect the unique experiences of different racial, ethnic, or income groups in the determination of—or response to—gender differences in health and health care.

ORGANIZATION OF THIS BOOK

This book is divided into four main sections. After an introduction documenting demographic, sociocultural and epidemiologic aspects of the gender difference, an overview of genetic and biological bases is presented, followed by a section on the influence of social roles and work on health and health care. The final section integrates biological and social explanations, providing conceptual and methodological evidence for linking morbidity and mortality data. The editors discuss the uncertainty of gender gap predictions in the Endnotes. Unanswered research questions and issues which require future research attention are highlighted.

Demographic, Sociocultural, and Epidemiological Perspectives

The introductory chapter by Dr. Constance Nathanson reviews demographic and sociocultural patterns in mortality differences between men and women, revealing how the gender gap is not static but differs throughout history, place, and social conditions. Drawing on cross-national data, the author discusses alternative explanations (biological, behavioral, and sociocultural) for understanding the gender differential in mortality and how it changes. The data presented illustrate the interrelationships among gender, social structure, and mortality. For example, gender differences in social class and smoking behaviors demonstrate the influence that sociocultural variables have on different mortality rates for men and women. In contrast to popular assumptions that changes in women's roles and activities will play a major role in the convergence of mortality rates, Nathanson cautiously concludes that any narrowing of the gender gap, which is only likely to occur in the upper socioeconomic status levels, will be accounted for by reductions in males' exposure to risk behavior and their increased health-promoting activities.

Further refining Nathanson's general sociodemographic overview of gender differences, the chapter by Dr. Deborah Wingard and Dr. Barbara Cohn focuses on variations in disease-specific sex–mortality ratios. An analysis of both vital statistics and population-based data from Alameda County, California, reveals that the sex ratios for health vary by age, disease, and outcome (morbidity and mortality). For example, heart disease mortality is greater for men than women, although this gender difference declines with age. In contrast, the gender difference in cancer mortality ranges from greater female mortality in young adults to greater male mortality in older adults. Such examinations of sex-, age-, and disease-specific risks elucidate the contribution of both biological and behavioral risk factors to the gender difference in health and longevity. A major methodological contribution of this chapter is the attention to the conceptualization and interpretation of sex ratios versus male–female differences in measuring both mortality and longevity. The examination of cancer and heart disease in both sets of data reveals the need to apply carefully the use of the sex ratio when investigating gender differences.

Genetic and Biological Bases

In an introductory chapter highlighting genetic and biological issues in aging research, Dr. David Smith and Dr. Huber Warner present an overview that examines the human longevity differential, and outlines the genotypic, hormonal and immunological differences between men and women that are thought to contribute to the gender gap. Setting the stage for the subsequent chapters that discuss these differences in more detail, they conclude by posing questions that can only be answered by future research.

Dr. James Neel examines the differential neonatal and early childhood survival of males and females. Although more males are conceived than females, male mortality is greater than that of females from birth through maturity. Neel examines various possible explanations for the greater in utero mortality of male fetuses, the slightly greater number of male births to female births and the higher male mortality rates in early life. The author also examines the impact of radiation exposure on the sex ratio. He concludes that genetic factors alone do not explain greater male mortality.

Dr. Stanley Gartler discusses the relevance of x-chromosome inactivation to the gender difference in longevity. He proposes that x-inactivation could contribute to the observed differential in at least three ways: the effect on the female of the embryology of x-inactivation; errors in the maintenance of the x-activation system; and the mosaic nature of the female leading to the possibility of somatic cell selection. He concludes that only the latter is likely to contribute substantially to the observed longevity difference.

Dr. William Hazzard examines metabolic processes that contribute to the sex differential in longevity. He argues that the gender difference in sex hormones leads to differences in the way men and women metabolize lipoproteins and that this, in turn, leads to a gender differential in the incidence of atherosclerosis. The resulting higher incidence of atherosclerosis and its complications in men contribute to the gender differential in longevity.

Dr. Marc Weksler brings together studies that examine whether females have a more vigorous immunological system, which protects them more effectively from disease, than do males. Specifically, he explores whether gender differences in human longevity are the result of women's greater immunological responsiveness. The author concludes that there is a very complex web of relationships among gender, age, and immunity.

The Impact of Social Roles on Health and Health Care Utilization

The differing social roles that men and women perform are often cited as major causes of the well-documented gender difference in health and longevity. In their chapter, Dr. Sonja McKinlay and colleagues take an in-depth look at the multiple roles held by middle-aged women (e.g., spouse, mother, caregiver, and worker) and the extent to which these roles are sources of stress. The authors are particularly interested in understanding the impact of employment status on women's physical and mental health. Drawing data from a large representative sample of community-residing women initially aged 45 to 55, these authors document that the majority of such women are performing multiple roles and that these roles may be sources of stress. However, work, per se, may actually be beneficial, even when added to other roles and responsibilities, and many of the reported stresses are surprisingly not translated into negative health outcomes. A major conclusion from this research is that more information is needed on how women manage multiple roles and the stresses that they cause. Longitudinal analyses, such as those conducted by McKinlay and colleagues, which differentiate multiple roles and health outcomes, can increase our understanding of the extent to which social roles and stresses impact men and women differentially.

Although there is a long history of research documenting differences in health care utilization between men and women, relatively little is known about gender differences across a wide range of health care services, especially for the very old. Dr. Cynthia Thomas and Dr. Howard Kelman examine the gender differences in health service utilization between men and women aged 65–98, examining hospitalization, physician visits, total ambulatory care, and health-related service use in a sample of respondents residing in the Bronx in New York City. In exploring whether differences in health status or psychosocial factors explain the higher hospitalization rates for elderly men relative to women, and the greater use of physician services for elderly women relative to men, they find that gender effects generally persist. Only for health-related services do gender differences disappear when simultaneously accounting for physical health, availability of economic resources, age, and mental health. Similar factors appear to be predicting utilization for both men and women, although variables vary somewhat in their importance for different utilization measures for men and women. This study shows the importance of examining gender differences in various types of health care utilization, since different patterns are found across types.

The Integration of Biological and Social Explanations: Linking Morbidity and Mortality Data

Women's higher rates of morbidity and use of therapeutic care in comparison to men's higher mortality rates are well documented. Using the Health in Detroit Study to examine the gender differences in health status and health behavior, Dr. Lois Verbrugge attempts to reconcile the seemingly contradictory sex differences in morbidity and mortality. Acquired risks, psychosocial factors, and health reporting behaviors are examined to explain women's higher morbidity. Interestingly, these risk factors do not consistently favor one sex over the other; for example, men are more likely to smoke and to be exposed to job hazards while women are more likely to suffer from stress, inactivity, and nonemployment. When risk factors for illness are controlled, the gender gap in morbidity narrows considerably. In some cases, controlling for risk factors reveals greater male rather than female morbidity. These results are compared to those obtained in recent analyses of sex mortality differences in three California sites. Verbrugge concludes that, while the different social experiences of men and women account for women's higher morbidity, men's excess mortality cannot be explained by social factors alone. Further interdisciplinary research is important for increasing our knowledge of how biological factors interact with social factors to explain male's underlying disadvantages in both morbidity and mortality.

Dr. Kenneth Manton in his chapter demonstrates how population-based models of morbidity, disability, and mortality can be developed into models that accurately reflect biological data and theory. An iterative process of model construction, empirical testing on population data, and evaluation of the model's performance are described. Manton uses these "biologically realistic population models" to examine sex differences in the age trajectories of mortality and morbidity in several different data sets, including the 1982–1984 National Long-Term Care Survey, Duke Longitudinal Survey and the Framingham Heart Study. This sophisticated conceptual and methodological presentation reveals the usefulness of models that are constructed to reflect biological insights in the analysis of population data. For example, these applications help us interpret sex differences in disability and mortality transitions. We see that the prevalence of disability is greater for females than for males, but that this difference is due more to females' greater survival at each impairment level than on sex differences in incidence levels—pointing to the importance of examining sex differences in the types of diseases causing disabilities. This chapter also adds valuable insights into the mechanisms by which risk factors affect mortality by addressing key issues such as: changes in risk factors with age, the effect of cohort specific differences, and the differential impact of risk factors on males versus females.

MARCIA G. ORY
HUBER R. WARNER

REFERENCES

Binstock, R. H., & Shanas, E. (Eds.). (1985). *Handbook of aging and the social sciences.* New York: Van Nostrand Reinhold.

Birren, J. E., & Schaie, K. W. (Eds.). (1985). *Handbook of the psychology of aging.* New York: Van Nostrand Reinhold.

Finch, C. E., & Schneider, E. L. (Eds.). (1985). *Handbook of the biology of aging.* New York: Van Nostrand Reinhold.

Ory, M. G., & Bond, K. (Eds.). (1989). *Aging and health care: Social science and policy perspectives.* London: Routledge.

Riley, M. W., Hess, B., & Bond, K. (Eds.). (1983). *Aging in Society: Selected Reviews of recent research.* Hillsdale, NJ: Lawrence Erlbaum Associates.

U.S. Senate Special Committee on Aging. (1988). *Aging America: Trends and predictions: 1987–1988.* Washington, DC: U.S. Government Printing Office.

I DEMOGRAPHIC, SOCIOCULTURAL, AND EPIDEMIOLOGIC PERSPECTIVES

1 The Gender–Mortality Differential in Developed Countries: Demographic and Sociocultural Dimensions

Constance A. Nathanson

This chapter describes the mortality differential between men and women and locates it in time and in geographic space. Several approaches are employed to identify factors that contribute to the sex mortality differential and to predict its future. The impact of social class and smoking behaviors are examined as an illustration of how sociocultural variables may influence the mortality rates of men and women. The more we know about sources of variation in the size of the "gender gap," the more informed will be our speculation concerning how its dimensions may change in the future.

EMERGENCE OF THE GENDER GAP

Higher female than male expectation of life at birth is associated, first of all, with a particular set of demographic and social conditions (i.e., conditions of low overall mortality and relatively high levels of social and economic development). Alan Lopez has defined the emergence of the gender gap as a four stage process; his formulation is shown in Table 1.1.

In the first "high mortality" stage, overall mortality is high and there is excess female mortality, particularly during childhood and in the childbearing years. This pattern was still present in India as recently as the early 1970s (United Nations Population Division, 1983; Bhatia, 1983). In the second stage of "intermediate mortality," corre-

Table 1.1 Stages in Gender-Mortality Transition

Stage	Transition
1. *High Mortality*	Excess female mortality especially in childhood and childbearing ages
2. *Intermediate Mortality*	Gender "crossover": female disadvantage disappears with development
3. *Low Mortality*	Stable or increased male mortality—rapid decline of female mortality
4. *Post-Transitional*	Hypothesized mortality convergence

Adapted from Alan D. Lopez, "Evolution of sex differentials in health and mortality," *IUSSP Newsletter* 32 (January–April, 1988).

sponding to a somewhat higher level of social and economic development, a "crossover" takes place from higher male to higher female expectation of life at birth. Most developing countries are now at this stage; it also describes the United States (and other Western countries) in the late nineteenth and early twentieth centuries. The third "low mortality" stage is, of course, familiar; it characterizes most developed countries today. In this stage, female mortality undergoes a rapid decline while male mortality remains relatively stable or even increases. Finally, Lopez postulates a "post-transitional" fourth stage of convergence in gender-mortality rates, an intriguing hypothesis that will be discussed in the last section of this chapter (Lopez, 1988).

First, however, it is useful to describe the parameters of the gender gap at stage three in somewhat greater detail, as this is the stage common to most industrialized countries. In all developed countries, the expectation of life for females exceeds that for males: the female advantage is 7 years in North America and 4 to 8 years in other developed countries (Torrey, Kinsella, & Taeuber, 1987). These figures reflect a steady widening of gender mortality differentials over the course of the twentieth century. This change is illustrated in Figure 1.1 based on data from the United States from 1900 to 1986. Because race has a substantial impact on the sex mortality differential in the United States, these data are shown by race. Between 1920 and 1970, the sex difference increased among whites by a factor of 6, and by a factor of 8 among blacks. Since 1970, however, the size of the gap in mortality has declined quite sharply among whites, and has begun to decline among blacks.

Figure 1.1 Sex difference in expectation of life at birth by race, United States, 1900–1986.

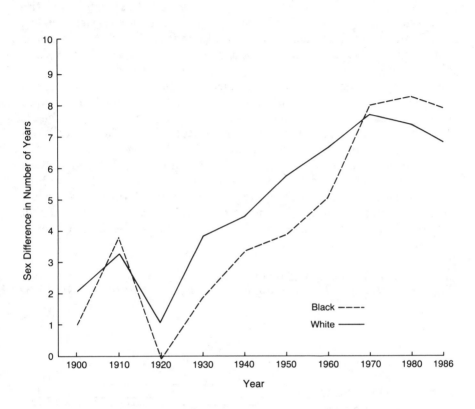

Sources: U.S. Department of Commerce, Bureau of the Census, *Historical Statistics of the United States, Colonial Times to 1970, Bicentennical Edition.* Part 1. Washington, D.C., 1975
U.S. Department of Health and Human Services, *Vital Statistics of the United States, Volume II—Mortality, 1986.* Part A. Hyattsville, Md., 1988.

More than one alternative pattern of change in the respective mortality rates of males and females could have produced the results shown in Figure 1.1. The patterns that have produced them (in the U.S. and in other developed countries as well) are more rapid improvement in female relative to male death rates and an increasing male disadvantage in death rates from the chronic conditions that are the leading causes of death in developed countries (Preston, 1976; Nathanson, 1984). The narrowing of the gender gap between 1970 and 1986 in the United States was due both to a decline in the rate of increase in females' expectation of life and to a sharp increase in the length of life that could be expected by males.

STRUCTURE AND VARIABILITY OF GENDER GAP

It is useful to think of the gender gap as having both *structure*—in the sense that certain groups in the population and certain causes of death contribute to it more than others—and (what is the other side of the same coin) *variability*—it is wider in some groups and under some circumstances than others. As Figure 1.2 shows, the largest cause-of-death contributor to the gender-mortality differential in developed countries is cardiovascular disease (the shaded bars show the principal disease processes under each cause-of-death): cardiovascular disease accounts for about 50% of the gender–mortality difference overall and for about 80% of the increase in the differential over time.[1]

Age groups, as well as causes of death, contribute differentially to the gender gap. Figure 1.3 refers to the United States and shows how the contributions of different age groups have changed over time, corresponding to change in the composition of causes. In the early 1900s, when the gap was relatively small (a little over 2 years), over

Figure 1.2 Contribution of leading causes of death to the average sex mortality differential in developed countries at ages 35 to 74, 1975–1978.

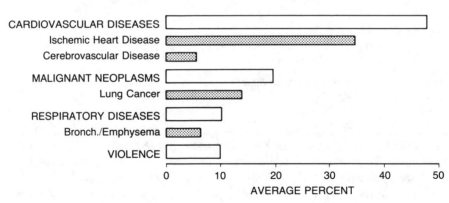

Source: From Alan D. Lopez, "The sex mortality differential in developed countries." In Alan D. Lopez and Lado T. Ruzicka (eds.), *Sex differentials in mortality,* pp. 53–120. Canberra: Australian National University, 1983.

50% of the difference was accounted for by deaths under the age of 5 years. At the most recent period, close to 40% of the gender-mortality differential is contributed to by deaths of individuals over 65.

As a preliminary specification, then, the explanatory problem posed by the gender gap might quite reasonably be narrowed to the problem of explaining gender-mortality differences in cardiovascular disease (principally ischemic heart disease) among persons of middle-age and older—or even further, perhaps, to the problem of explaining the slow rate of improvement in mortality rates from these conditions of older males.

In addition to the structural perspective outlined above, a second approach to the development of explanatory hypotheses is the identification of sets of circumstances under which the phenomenon in question is present to a greater or a lesser degree. The gender gap lends itself to this approach, because not only *among* but *within* developed countries its size is remarkably variable. Figure 1.4 describes the variation among countries. To provide some perspective, the three bars that correspond to the average gap of 6.4 years (in 1975–1978) have been shaded and the entire 33 countries have been divided into approximate quartiles—the gender gap is, for example, very large in

Figure 1.3 Age components of the sex differential in life expectancy at birth, United States, 1900–1978.

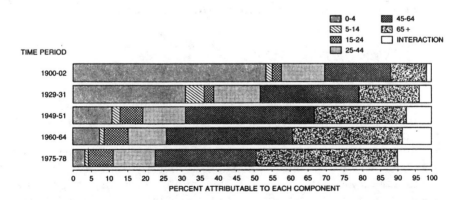

Source: From Alan D. Lopez, "The sex mortality differential in developed countries." In Alan D. Lopez and Lado T. Ruzicka (eds.), *Sex differentials in mortality*, pp. 53–120. Canberra: Australian National University, 1983.

the USSR and in Finland (and relatively large in the United States); it is very small in Japan and in Greece. To complicate this picture further, it is important to point out that *among* these developed countries, all of which fall into the third "low mortality" stage of the gender-mortality transition, there is no simple relationship between the level of mortality and the size of the gender gap. The United States and Greece, for example, have identical crude mortality rates (and very similar age distributions) but the U.S. has one of the largest gender gaps and Greece one of the smallest. In an attempt to further specify the dimensions of cross-national variation in the size of the gender gap, data are presented in Figure 1.5 comparing the relative contributions of male and female mortality to the gender gap in "large gap" and "small gap" countries. The vertical lines in Figure 1.5 represent the average gender gap (6.4) years for 35 developed countries, based on the expectation of life at birth.[2] Horizontal bars represent the amount that each sex's "excess" or "deficit" mortality contributes to each country's departure from the overall average gap in life expectation. Very generally, countries with large gaps tend to be characterized by excess male mortality and/or substantial "deficits" in female mortality. Small gap countries, with the exceptions of Japan and Greece, tend to have markedly above average female mortality. The cases of Japan and Greece are clearly unique; their experience deserves more detailed investigation by students of sex mortality differentials.

In addition to variation among countries, the size of the gender gap varies widely within countries. "Social class" represents one of the most uniform as well as the most intriguing of these variations. This source of variation will be explored in greater detail after a somewhat broader perspective on the nature of the explanatory problems presented by gender differences in mortality is presented.

PROBLEMS OF EXPLANATION

One of the most striking facts about research in gender-mortality differences is its cross-disciplinary nature. It is hardly suprising to find that disciplinary orientation influences rather powerfully *what* about the gender gap is seen to require explanation—the biologically oriented scholar emphasizes the constancy of this differential, the social scientist its variation—and *where* investigators are likely to look for explanatory variables. It is the uniquely protean quality of sex as a conceptual category that allows the scholars to see in it that for which their training has prepared them to look: the biologist sees

Figure 1.4 Sex differential in life expentancy at birth, developed countries, 1975–1978.

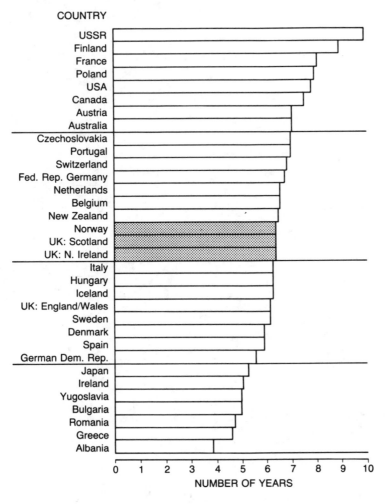

Source: From Alan D. Lopez, "The sex mortality differential in developed countries." In Alan D. Lopez and Lado T. Ruzicka (eds.), *Sex differentials in mortality*, pp. 53–120. Canberra: Australian National University, 1983.

hormones and chromosomes; the epidemiologist, risk factors; and the sociologist, social roles and structural constraints. While this division of labor is not expected to change, the different perspectives need not be contradictory.

Figure 1.5 Components of departure from average life expectancy due to deviations in male and female mortality, developed countries, 1975–1978.

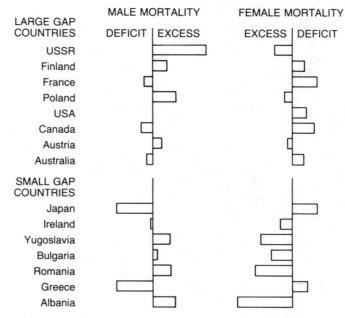

Source: From Alan D. Lopez, "The sex mortality differential in developed countries." In Alan D. Lopez and Lado T. Ruzicka (eds.), *Sex differentials in mortality*, pp. 53–120. Canberra: Australian National University, 1983.

The Social Science Perspective

The observation of variation in the size of the gender gap—over time, across countries and cultures, and according to social class, religion, marital status, and employment—has led to the questioning of *exclusively* biological theories of causation and to the generation of hypotheses that emphasize primarily social and behavioral rather than biological causal variables. Even if it were true that females possessed an innate biological advantage, the fact of variation in the *size* of that advantage (remembering that its size is a function of *both* sexes' mortality rates) would still require explanation.

Toward a Multidisciplinary Explanatory Model

Explanation at the biological level, then, does not preclude explanation at the sociocultural level, nor does establishing the importance of sociocultural variables mean that biological variables can safely be ignored. There is some tendency in both social and epidemiological research on mortality to treat *all but* the major variable of interest (whether that variable be social network density, income level, alcohol use, or personality type) as what are known as "confounders"—noise in the system that prevents a clear test of the investigator's central hypothesis. A more complex, but ultimately more correct, explanatory model would treat biological (as well as other intrapersonal) risk factors as *part of* the system and as factors that mediate the impact of broader social influences on mortality.

Causes of the Gender Gap

In Table 1.2, hypothetical "causes" of the gender gap have been divided into three very broad groups: biological, behavioral, and sociocultural. The "biological" genetic and hormonal hypotheses are considered in detail in other chapters of this book (see for example chapters by Smith, Gartler, Hazzard, and Weksler). Here, attention will be drawn to the two large classes of nonbiological "causes" that have been proposed: behavioral (or individual level) causes—for example, individual differences in smoking behavior—and sociocultural (or group level) causes—for example, differences between countries in economic modernization or in the status of women.

A brief review of the behavioral hypotheses begins with an explanation of the gender gap in terms of male–female differences in exposure to acquired mortality risks. In developed countries attention has fo-

Table 1.2 Causes of the Gender Gap

I.   Biological: Genetic/Hormonal

II.   Behavioral (Individual level)
      1. Differences in exposure to acquired mortality risks
      2. Differences in self-protective behavior
      3. Differences in psycho/social stress

III. Sociocultural (Group level)
      1. Position of women
      2. Position of men

cused primarily on differential participation in potentially risky modes of behavior such as smoking, drinking, driving, and violence (Nathanson, 1977; Harrison, 1978; Ortmeyer, 1979; Waldron, 1983). However, with the exception of cigarette smoking, sex differences in overt risk-taking behaviors do not appear to account for more than a small proportion of the sex-mortality differential. Behavioral hypotheses also explain the gender gap by referring to differences between males and females in the probability of engaging in *self-protective* behavior. Although women in Western countries do make greater use of preventive and curative health services, to date there is no direct evidence that these behaviors have a significant effect on gender differences in mortality. Finally, behavioral hypotheses suggest that men may be exposed to relatively higher levels of social and/or psychological stress and that this is at least partially responsible for the gender gap (see Chapter 11). There has been considerable speculation that higher frequency of the Type A behavior pattern among men was associated with the gender gap in mortality, but the evidence supporting this notion is quite weak. (Literature on which the foregoing statements are based is reviewed in detail in Nathanson, 1984).

Sociocultural variables include empirical indicators of individuals' positions in the social structure (e.g., marital status and social class) as well as broader structural indices such as urbanization or the percentage of women employed outside the home. The subheadings, "position of women," "position of men," reflect the fact that analysts tend to interpret these variables in terms of their implications for the relative ease or difficulty of men's and women's positions in the larger society (e.g., marriage is good for men, not so good [relatively speaking] for women; urbanization is good for women, not so good for men (Preston, 1976; Pampel & Zimmer, 1987). It is through their influence on gender roles or positions that sociocultural variables are presumed to influence mortality. The example of social class as a particular group level (or, in sociological terms, "structural") variable will be used in the next section to illustrate some of the specific mechanisms by which variables at the structural level may affect the mortality of individual men and women.

STRUCTURAL INFLUENCES ON MORTALITY PATTERNS

There is a substantial body of data showing that in developed countries mortality is inversely related to measures of social class: the higher the class (or occupational or income) level, the lower the mortality (Antonovsky, 1967; Kitagawa & Hauser, 1973; United Nations, 1982).

However, much of the relevant research has focused on males; recent studies from at least eight developed countries (United States, Canada, Great Britain, Finland, Denmark, Norway, France, Japan) present evidence that social class effects are less pronounced among females (Araki & Murata, 1986; Desplanques, 1984; Koskenvuo, Kaprio, Lonnqvist & Sarna, 1986; Lynge, 1981; Millar, 1983; Passanante, 1983; Rose & Marmot, 1981; Valkonen & Sauli, 1981; Wingard, Suarez, & Barrett-Conner, 1983; Yeracaris & Kim, 1978).

Gender, Social Class, and Mortality Interactions

Data to illustrate the interrelationships among gender, social class, and mortality suggested by these studies are shown in Figure 1.6. This figure is based on the Canadian data described by Millar (1983); it gives the number of years of life expected at birth by gender and by the income level of the census tract in which the decedent resided. These data demonstrate two important points. First, they show that sex-mortality differences are over $1\frac{1}{2}$ times larger at the lowest than at the highest income level. Second, they show that this difference is due primarily to variation in *male's* rather than in *female's* expectation of life. Figure 1.7, drawn from the same paper, shows gender by income level gradient for age-standardized mortality rates specifically from ischemic heart disease; the rates are for persons 35 to 64 years old. Again, the size of the difference at the lowest income level is about $1\frac{1}{2}$ times that at the upper level; the gender-income level interactive effect is caused by the marked influence of income level on *male* mortality rates. Parallel findings have been reported from Great Britain, France, and the Scandanavian countries: uniformly, the data show a larger gender gap at lower than at higher social class levels *produced by* a steeper social class gradient for men than for women.

There is some evidence that the gender–social class–mortality interaction described is of relatively recent origin, possibly because social class effects on *male* mortality in developed countries have been increasing as total mortality has declined. An analysis of socioeconomic status differences in mortality based on data from the United States concluded that decreases in mortality were more likely to be experienced by members of higher socioeconomic classes, that relative increases in mortality were most likely to be experienced by lower socioeconomic classes, and that both of these effects were more pronounced for males than females (Yeracaris & Kim, 1978). Parallel trends have been observed in Great Britain. Marmot and McDowall (1978) reported a reversal of the social class gradient for heart disease among men between the years 1931 and 1971. In the earlier period,

Figure 1.6 Expectation of life at birth by income level and gender, Canada, 1971.

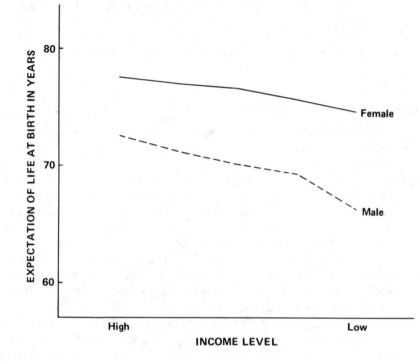

Source: From W. A. Millar, Sex differentials in mortality by income level in urban Canada. *Canadian Journal of Public Health, 74,* (September/October, 1983).

upper-class men had the higher rates; by 1961, rates were higher for lower-class men in all age groups. No change was noted in the social class gradient for women. A more recent analysis comparing 1970–1972 with 1979–1983 data showed a continuing increase in the relative mortality disadvantage of manual relative to nonmanual workers (for all causes of death), but the effect was present for women as well as men (Marmot & McDowall, 1986). Finally, Pell and Fayerweather (1985) compared trends in the incidence of myocardial infarction among blue- and white-collar DuPont Company employees from 1957 through 1983. Among males, there was a decline in age-adjusted incidence for both categories of employees, but the amount of the decline among white-collar was double that of blue-collar workers. No consistent trends in incidence of myocardial infarction were observed among female employees.

Figure 1.7 Mortality rates for ischemic heart disease by income level and gender, Canada, 1971.

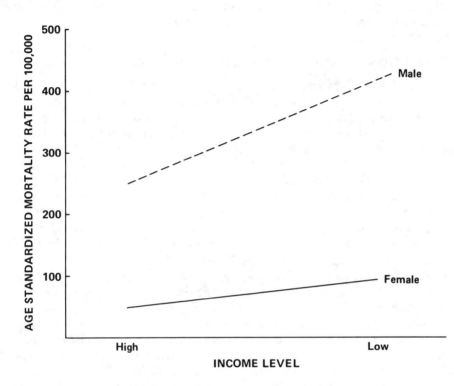

Source: From W. A. Millar, "Sex differentials in mortality by income level in urban Canada." *Canadian Journal of Public Health, 74,* (September/October, 1983).

Given the difficult methodological problems that attend research on mortality and social class (United Nations, 1982; Fox & Goldblatt, 1982; Bloor, Samphier, & Prior, 1987), the trends described should be treated as provisionally established at best. Nevertheless, they are useful as the basis for further elaboration of one possible explanatory approach to the gender gap.

The social class data presented suggest an intriguing (and deliberately overstated and oversimplified) hypothesis: the gender gap in developed countries is increasingly accounted for by the divergent mortality rates of blue-collar men. In other words, the sex differential in mortality is as much a product of social class as of gender. This hypothesis can be evaluated in a *very* preliminary way by examining its compatibility with the distribution by gender and social class of known behavioral risk factors for mortality. For example, cigarette smoking can be conceived of as a pathway, or intervening variable, that mediates between a set of social circumstances defined by gender and social class and a biological outcome, mortality.

Social Class Differences in Cigarette Smoking

Social class differences in smoking behavior do, in fact, correspond quite closely to observed gender–social class–mortality relationships. Data presented in Figure 1.8 are based on national samples of the United States population and show the percentages of those who are current smokers by gender and educational level for three years separated by intervals of approximately ten years. In all three time periods, men with lower levels of education have been substantially more likely to smoke than either better educated men or women. The difference between men's and women's smoking patterns *within* the two least well educated categories is particularly sharp in the earliest time period, surely the most relevant for current mortality rates. By contrast, the smoking behavior of college-educated men and women was quite similar even in 1964 and has tended to become increasingly similar over time, due primarily to decreases in smoking by better-educated men. More recent evidence of the gender–social class interactive effect on smoking behavior (in which occupation rather than education is used to index socioeconomic status) is provided by the data shown in Figure 1.9. This figure shows percentages of current smokers among individuals aged 20 and over in 1970, 1978 to 1980, and 1985. In 1970 these percentages were virtually identical, and equally low, among blue and white collar women and white collar men; the divergent behavior of blue collar men, among whom over 50% were current smokers, is very clear. Over time, however, as the prevalence of smoking among men (both white and blue collar) has declined more rapidly than among women, gender differences in smoking within the blue-collar group, although still present, have become less marked. Parallel data from Great Britain are presented in Figure 1.10. They show an almost identical pattern of change between 1972 and 1982 in the gender–social class distribution of smoking to that described for the United States by Figure 1.9.

Thus, the distribution of a major mortality risk factor, smoking, has a pattern of interaction with gender and social class similar to the pattern of mortality rates recently observed in several developed countries. And the *illustrative* model presented to explain the gender gap now has four variables: gender and social class as exogenous

Figure 1.8 Percentages of current smokers by educational level and gender, United States, 1964, 1975, and 1983.

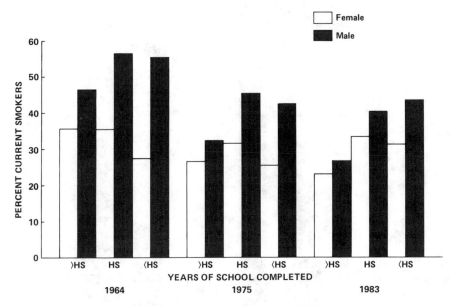

Source: U.S. Department of Health, Education, and Welfare. *Smoking and Health: A Report of the Surgeon General.* DHEW Publication No. (PHS) 79-50066, Washington, DC. 1979.

C. A. Scheonborn & B. H. Cohen: Trends in smoking, alchohol consumption, and other health practices among U.S. adults, 1977 and 1983. *Advance Data from Vital and Health Statistics,* No. 118 (Supplement), DHHS Pub. No. (PHS) 86-1250, Public Health Service, Hyattsville, MD., June 30, 1986.

independent variables; smoking as an intervening variable or mechanism; and mortality as the outcome variable. (The data that have been presented do not, of course, demonstrate that smoking *is* the most important intervening variable in accounting for gender–social class effects on mortality, or that the suggested model is a correct representation of reality. The model is presented to illustrate an approach to explanation rather than as an explanation itself.)

IMPORTANCE OF SOCIAL AND BIOLOGICAL INFLUENCES ON "RISKY BEHAVIORS"

The purpose in presenting these data on smoking patterns was not to demonstrate yet again the lethal consequences of smoking. Quite the contrary. The explanation of differential mortality requires us to take

Figure 1.9 Prevalence of cigarette smoking by occupation and gender among individuals aged 16 and over, Great Britain, 1972 and 1982.

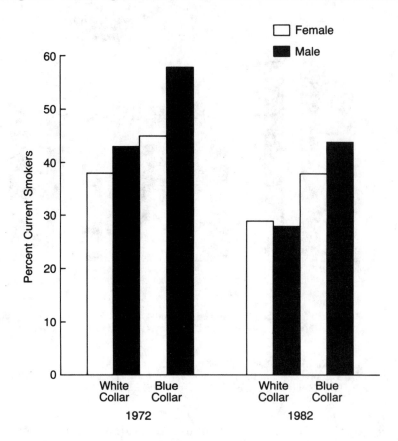

Source: M. G. Marmot and M. D. McDowall, "Mortality decline and widening social inequalities," *The Lancet*, August 2, 1986.

account not only of risky life-styles but of the social structures in which those life-styles are engendered and maintained. The latter as much as the former are "causes" of mortality. The data shown in Figures 1.8 through 1.10 reveal a striking pattern of change over time in the *social location* of smoking. During a period of highly visible and publicly sanctioned attention to its deleterious health consequences, smoking has declined differentially by gender and social class, becoming increasingly concentrated among blue collar men and, to a slightly lesser

Figure 1.10 Prevalence of cigarette smoking by occupation and gender among individuals over 20, United States, 1970, 1978 to 1980, and 1985.

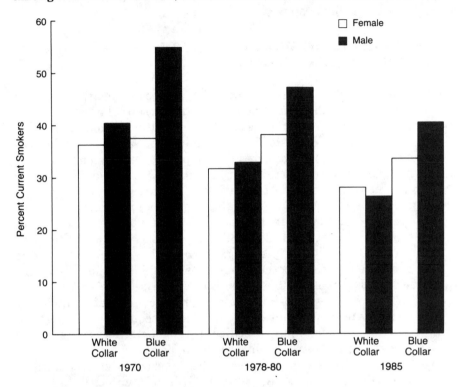

Source: U.S. Department of Health and Human Services, *Reducing the Health Consequences of Smoking: 25 Years of Progress. Report of the Surgeon General, 1989.*

extent, blue collar women. Initiation, persistence in, and discontinuation of this "risky" behavior cannot be understood apart from the social context in which this behavior occurs. A complete model to explain variation in the size of the gender gap by social class (insofar as the gap is explained by smoking patterns) would require not only that biological links be established between cigarette smoking and mortality (as has been done) and that behavioral links be established between gender and cigarette smoking, but also that links based in sociological theory be established between social class structure and the gender role dimensions that support or discourage cigarette smoking. These latter sociocultural variables are causes of mortality of importance equal to that of individual behavior or biological variation. It should be emphasized that the approach described is equally applicable to understanding the role of other potentially important life-style links between gender, social class, and mortality: diet and recreational exercise patterns, for example.

CONVERGENCE IN MORTALITY RATES: CHANGES IN MEN'S BEHAVIOR

What can be said about Alan Lopez's fourth "post-transitional" stage in the gender-mortality transition (see Table 1.1) and the hypothesis of mortality convergence? Analyses of the sociocultural dimension of the gender gap have tended to focus on the positive or negative consequences of social arrangements for the position of women or men in society. When it comes to prediction, popular as well as some scholarly attention has focused almost exclusively on current and prospective changes in the position of women: convergence in mortality rates has been predicted on the grounds of increased participation by women in extrafamilial activities associated (the hypothesis runs) with the adoption of risky "male" life-styles (e.g., Lewis & Lewis, 1977). There is little evidence for this hypothesis and considerable evidence against it (reviewed in Nathanson, 1984; see also Pampel & Zimmer, 1987). An alternative hypothesis posits that convergence in gender mortality rates is likely to come about, if at all, as a consequence of changes in the behavior of *men*. More specifically, gender differentials in industrialized societies may converge at upper socioeconomic status levels due primarily to the presence at these levels of a set of conditions that, first, reduces males' exposure, and possibly vulnerability, to a variety of health risks *and*, second, increases the probability of behavioral change in response to health education. Convergence at lower status levels appears less likely. However, given the long lag time between initiation of risky behaviors and their lethal consequences, as well as the strong possibility of social change in cohort behaviors and survival patterns over time, any predictions for the future should be regarded with extreme caution.

NOTES

1. Summary data on developed countries presented in this chapter are based on analyses carried out by Alan Lopez and reported at a conference on sex–mortality differentials held in 1981 at Canberra, Australia under the sponsorship of the Australian National University, the United Nations, and the World Health Organization. This

work was published in 1983 (Alan D. Lopez, *"The sex mortality differential in developed countries,"* pp. 53–120 in Alan D. Lopez and Lado T. Ruzicka, eds., *Sex differentials in mortality.* Canberra: Australian National University, 1983). I know of no more recent work comparable to Dr. Lopez's in breadth of country coverage and range of comparative analyses. With respect to the definition of developed countries, Dr. Lopez states that classification "will adhere to the United Nations definition and be taken to include the United States of America, Canada, Australia, New Zealand, Japan, the Union of Soviet Socialist Republics and all regions of Europe" (55).

2. The calculations on which this figure is based are reported in Alan D. Lopez (1983). Data are for 1975–1977/1978 with two exceptions. USSR data are for 1971–1972 and Albanian data are from 1969–1970.

REFERENCES

Antonovsky, A. (1967). Social class, life expectancy, and overall mortality. *Milbank Memorial Fund Quarterly, 45,* 31–73.

Araki, S., & K. Murata. (1986). Social life factors affecting the mortality of total Japanese population. *Social Science and Medicine, 23,* 1168–1169.

Bhatia, S. (1983). Traditional practices affecting female health and survival: evidence from countries of South Asia. In A. D. Lopez & L. T. Ruzicka (eds.), *Sex differentials in mortality,* pp. 165–177. Canberra: Australian National University Press.

Bloor, M., Samphier, M., & Prior, L. (1987). Artefact explanations of inequalities in health: an assessment of the evidence. *Sociology of Health and Illness, 9,* 231–264.

Desplanques, G. (1984). Le mortalite selon le milieu social en France. *Socioeconomic Differential Mortality in Industrialized Societies.* Vol. 3. United Nations Population Division (New York)/World Health Organization (Geneva)/Committee for International Cooperation in National Research in Demography (Paris).

Fox, A. J., & Goldblatt, P. O. (1982). *Longitudinal study: Socioeconomic mortality differentials.* Office of Population Censuses and Surveys, Series LS, No. 1. London: Her Majesty's Stationery Office.

Harrison, J. (1978). Warning: the male sex role may be dangerous to your health. *Journal of Social Issues, 34,* 65–86.

Kitagawa, E. M., & Hauser, P. M. (1973). *Differential mortality in the United States: A study in socioeconomic epidemiology.* Cambridge, MA: Harvard University Press.

Koskenvuo, M., Kaprio, J., Lonnqvist, J., & Sarna, S. (1986). Social factors and the gender difference in mortality. *Social Science and Medicine, 23,* 605–609.

Lewis, C. E., & Lewis, R. N. (1977). The potential impact of sexual equality on health. *New England Journal of Medicine, 297,* 863–869.

Lopez, A. D. (1983). The sex mortality differential in developed countries. In A. D. Lopez & L. T. Ruzicka (eds.), *Sex differentials in mortality,* pp. 53–120. Canberra: Australian National University Press.

Lopez, A. D. (1988). Evolution of sex differentials in health and mortality. *IUSSP Newsletter,* 32 (January–April).

Lopez, A. D., & Ruzicka, L. T. (eds.). (1983). *Sex differentials in mortality.* Canberra: Australian National University Press.

Lynge, E. (1981). Occupation mortality in Norway, Denmark, and Finland. *Socioeconomic differential mortality in industrialized societies.* Vol. 1. United Nations Population Division (New York)/World Health Organization (Geneva)/Committee for International Cooperation in National Research in Demography (Paris).

Marmot, M. G. & McDowall, M. E. (1986). Mortality decline and widening social inequalities. *The Lancet,* 8501 (August 2), 274–276.

Millar, W. H. (1983). Sex differences in mortality by income level in urban Canada. *Canadian Journal of Public Health, 74,* 329–334.

Nathanson, C. A. (1977). Sex roles as variables in preventive health behavior. *Journal of Community Health, 3,* 142–155.

Nathanson, C. A. (1984). Sex differences in mortality. *Annual Review of Sociology, 10,* 191–213.

Ortmeyer, L. E. (1979). Females' natural advantages? Or, the unhealthy environment of males? The status of sex mortality differentials. *Women and Health, 4,* 121–133.

Passannante, M. (1983). *Female labor force participation and mortality.* Doctoral Dissertation, Johns Hopkins University, Baltimore, MD.

Pampel, F. C., & Zimmer, C. (1987). Female labor force activity and the sex differential in mortality: comparisons across developed countries, 1950–1975. Presented at the annual meeting of the Population Association of America, Chicago, IL.

Pell, S., & Fayerweather, W. E. (1985). Trends in the incidence of myocardial infarction and in associated mortality and morbidity in a large employed population, 1957–1983. *The New England Journal of Medicine, 312,* 1005–1011.

Preston, S. H. (1976). *Mortality patterns in national populations with special reference to recorded causes of death.* New York: Academic Press.

Rose, G., & Marmot, M. G. (1981). Social class and coronary heart disease. *British Heart Journal, 45,* 13–19.

Torrey, B. B., Kinsella, K., & Taeuber, C. M. (1987). *An aging world.* International Population Reports Series P-95, No. 78, Washington, DC: U.S. Bureau of the Census.

United Nations Department of International Economic and Social Affairs. (1982). *Levels and trends of mortality since 1950.* (ST/ESA/SER/A/7). New York: United Nations.

United Nations Population Division. (1983). Patterns of sex differentials in mortality in less developed countries. In A. D. Lopez & L. T. Ruzicka (eds.), *Sex differentials in mortality,* pp. 7–32. Canberra: Australian National University Press.

U.S. Department of Commerce, Bureau of the Census. (1975). *Historical statistics of the United States, colonial times to 1970, Bicentennial Edition.* Part 1. Washington, D.C.

U.S. Department of Health, Education, and Welfare. (1979). *Smoking and health: A report of the surgeon general.* DHEW Publication No. (PHS) 79-50066, Washington, DC: U.S. Government Printing Office.

U.S. Department of Health and Human Services. (1989). *Reducing the health consequences of smoking: 25 Years of progress.* Report of the Surgeon General.

U.S. Department of Health and Human Services. (1988). *Vital statistics of the United States, Volume II—Mortality, 1986.* Part A. Hyattsville, MD.

Valkonen, T., & Sauli, H. (1981). Socioeconomic differential mortality in Finland. *Socioeconomic differential mortality in industrialized societies.* Vol. 1. United Nations Population Division (New York)/World Health Organization (Geneva)/Committee for International Cooperation in National Research in Demography (Paris).

Waldron, I. (1983). Sex differences in human mortality: the role of genetic factors. *Social Science and Medicine, 17,* 321–333.

Wingard, D. L., Suarez, L., & Barrett-Conner, E. (1983). The sex differential in mortality for all causes and ischemic heart disease. *American Journal of Epidemiology, 117,* 165–172.

Yeracaris, C. A., & Kim, J. H. (1978). Socioeconomic differentials in selected causes of death. *American Journal of Public Health, 68,* 342–351.

2 Variations in Disease-Specific Sex Morbidity and Mortality Ratios in the United States

Deborah L. Wingard
Barbara A. Cohn

This chapter will focus on variations within the gender difference in longevity by describing sex differentials for mortality by age, time, and cause observed in both United States vital statistics data and data from a long-term population-based cohort, the Alameda County Study. In addition, variations in sex differentials for morbidity in the Alameda County Study will also be presented. These data illustrate the remarkable heterogeneity of sex differentials in health. By studying these variations in sex differentials in health, we may gain insights into the complex relationships between biological, behavioral, and psychosocial factors that influence health and longevity.

METHODOLOGIC ISSUES AND INTERPRETATION

The sex differential in mortality has generally been measured by the ratio or difference of male and female mortality rates (M/F, M–F) or life expectancy (F/M, F–M). The use of ratios or differences provides different information (Wingard, 1984; Verbrugge, 1980): ratios assess the relative differential in male and female mortality; differences assess the magnitude of the differential. Differences are useful for determining the contribution of various causes of death to the overall sex mortality differential and for comparing the actual number of deaths that occur among men and women. Ratios are better, however, when assessing changes in sex differentials in mortality over time, as differences will reflect both changes in sex differentials in mortality and changes in the risk of death over time. Similarly, ratios may be preferred when comparing sex differentials for specific causes of death for the purposes of generating hypotheses about disease etiology, because cause-specific sex ratios are independent of the proportion of death accounted for by each cause. Table 2.1 illustrates this point, showing that sex differences by cause may depend on the frequency of the cause, while sex ratios may not. In this chapter, sex ratios will be presented as measures of the sex differential by cause, although interesting aspects of sex differences comparisons will also be noted. Comparison of both differences and ratios allows the fullest assessment of the sex differential in mortality.

Whether using differences or ratios to examine the sex differential in mortality, age differences in the population must also be considered. Women live longer than men, so the female population considered as a whole is older than the male population. Therefore, mortality rates need to be age-adjusted or examined in age-specific categories. Comparisons of life-expectancy automatically adjust for differences in the age distribution of men and women.

UNITED STATES VITAL STATISTICS DATA

In the United States, sex mortality differentials, as measured by the ratio of male to female age-adjusted mortality rates, have favored women throughout this century (Wingard, 1984; Hazzard, 1986; Verbrugge, 1980; Johnson, 1977; Retherford, 1975). This differential in mortality rates increased steadily from 1.1 in 1900 to 1.8 in 1980 (Wingard, 1984). By 1980, the age-adjusted death rates in the United States were 777 deaths per 100,000 for men and 433 deaths per 100,000 for women, while the estimated life expectancy at birth was 70.0 years for men and 77.5 years for women (NCHS, 1983).

The male excess for mortality in 1980 was observed at every age,

Table 2.1 Comparison of Sex Mortality Differences and Ratios for Causes with Higher vs. Lower Frequencies of Occurrence

	Mortality rate/100		Sex difference (M/F)	Sex ratio (M/F)
	Males	Females		
Cause A	20	10	10	2
Cause B	10	5	5	2
Cause C	5	2.5	2.5	2

although the ratio of male to female rates varied with age (Wingard, 1984; NCHS, 1983). The sex ratio for mortality was greatest between ages 15 to 34, and declined thereafter, particularly after age 65 (Wingard, 1984; NCHS, 1983). However, in terms of sheer numbers, the sex differential was most dramatic in the older ages where the difference in death rates was greater.

In the United States in 1980, the age-adjusted mortality rate for each of the 12 leading causes of death was higher for men than women (NCHS, 1983). As can be seen in Table 2.2, the sex ratio varied from 3.9 (homicide) to 1.0 (diabetes). Those causes with a nearly two-fold or greater difference in the sex ratio listed in decreasing order were homicide, lung cancer, suicide, chronic obstructive pulmonary disease, accidents, cirrhosis of the liver, and heart disease. Many of these causes have a strong behavioral component: violent and traumatic deaths (homicide, suicide, accidents), smoking-related diseases (lung cancer, chronic obstructive pulmonary disease, heart disease), and alcohol-related diseases (cirrhosis, accidents).

As can be seen in Table 2.2, those causes of death that show the largest sex *ratios* are not among the three leading causes of death. To determine which causes of death contribute most to the sex differential in total mortality for various age groups, sex *differences* in cause-specific mortality rates can be employed. From such analysis, it has been determined that accidents are the main contributor to the peak in the sex mortality differential at younger ages, whereas heart disease is the main contributor to the differential at older ages (Retherford, 1975; Waldron, 1974).

Figure 2.1 illustrates that secular trends in the sex ratio vary by cause. Between 1950 and 1980, the male excess of lung cancer mortality in the United States demonstrated a particularly dramatic decline, due primarily to greater increases in lung cancer mortality rates for women (NCHS, 1986). In contrast, the sex differential in ischemic heart disease mortality remained relatively stable during this period, although mortality for both sexes has been declining since 1968 (NCHS, 1986).

Figures 2.2 and 2.3 illustrate that variations in the sex mortality ratios by age differ by cause as well (NCHS, 1986). In 1980, the sex mortality ratio for heart disease declined steeply with increasing age (Figure 2.2). In contrast, the sex mortality ratio for cancer increased with age, although the increase with age for cancer mortality was not as steep as the decline with age for heart disease mortality. The sex mortality ratio for suicide in 1980 showed a u-shaped relationship with age, with the lowest male excess between 35 and 54, a larger male excess under age 35 and the greatest male excess after age 64 (Figure

Table 2.2 Sex Mortality Ratios and Sex-Specific Mortality Rates for the Twelve Leading Causes of Death, United States, 1980

Cause of death [ICDA Nos.]	Sex ratio (M/F)	Age-adjusted mortality rate (per 100,000)[a]		Rank[b]
		Males	Females	
Homicide [E960–E978]	3.9	17.4	4.5	11
Suicide [E950–E959]	3.3	18.0	5.4	10
Chronic obstructive pulmonary disease (COPD) [490–496]	2.9	26.1	8.9	5
Accidents (including motor vehicle accidents) [E800–E949]	2.9	64.0	21.8	4
Cirrhosis of the liver [571]	2.2	17.1	7.9	8
Diseases of the heart [390–398, 402, 404–429]	2.0	280.4	140.3	1
Pneumonia and Influenza [480–487]	1.8	17.4	9.8	6
Cancer [140–208][c]	1.5	165.5	109.2	2
Atherosclerosis [440]	1.3	6.6	5.0	9
Certain causes in infancy [760–779]	1.3	11.1	8.7	12
Cerebrovascular diseases [430–438]	1.2	44.9	37.6	3
Diabetes mellitus [250]	1.0	10.2	10.0	7

Calculated from data in National Center for Health Statistics (1983).
[a]Direct age-adjusted to the 1940 total U.S. population.
[b]Rank based on number of deaths.
[c]Lung cancer [140–149] had a sex ratio of 3.4.

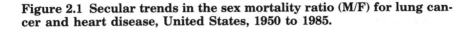

**Figure 2.1 Secular trends in the sex mortality ratio (M/F) for lung can-
cer and heart disease, United States, 1950 to 1985.**

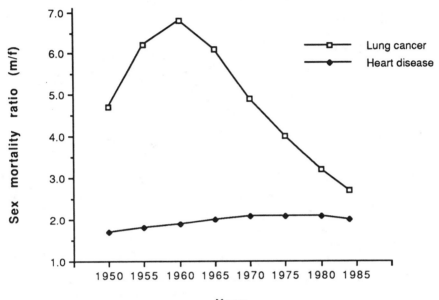

Based on mortality rates age-adjusted to the 1940 total U.S. population. Calculated from
data in National Center for Health Statistics (NCHS, 1986).

2.3). In contrast, the male excess in the sex mortality ratio for homicide
was large and constant up to age 64, declining thereafter.

These variations in the sex ratio within cause and between causes
may be the result of both biologic and behavioral differences between
men and women that vary by age. For example, variations in the sex
ratio with age may reflect hormonal changes in women due to menarche and the menopause. Or they may reflect age-specific differences in
behavioral risk factors (i.e., men may begin using cigarettes or alcohol
at a younger age). Alternatively, variations in the sex ratio with age
may reflect sex differences in cohort exposures. For example, for cancer
mortality the higher sex ratios at older ages (Figure 2.2) reflect the
larger sex difference in smoking behavior for birth cohorts born prior
to 1911 (USDHHS, 1980).

Figure 2.2 Age-specific sex mortality ratio (M/F) for cancer and heart disease, United States, 1980.

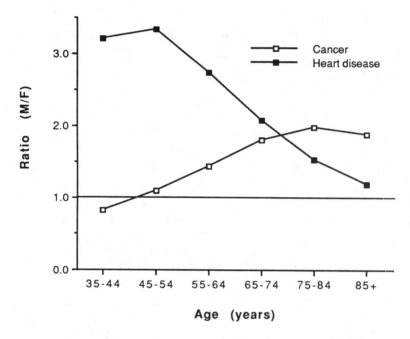

Calculated from data in National Center for Health Statistics (NCHS, 1986).

THE ALAMEDA COUNTY STUDY

Population-based cohort studies provide additional information concerning the heterogeneity of sex differentials in health. Unlike vital statistics data, cohort data track the morbidity and mortality experience of a specific cohort through time. This permits control of extraneous factors such as age structure, place, and time, which can influence sex differentials for morbidity and mortality. In addition, cohort studies often have information on behavioral and social risk factors for health outcomes that can be used to understand the contribution of these factors to sex differences in health.

This section focuses on sex differentials in health in a representative population sample of Alameda, California surveyed in 1965 and fol-

Figure 2.3 Age-specific sex mortality ratio (M/F) for homicide and suicide, United States, 1980.

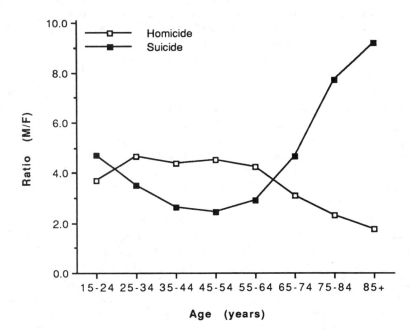

Calculated from data in National Center for Health Statistics (NCHS, 1986).

lowed for mortality through 1983 by the Human Population Laboratory, of the California Department of Health Services (Wingard, Cohn, Kaplan, Cirillo, & Cohen, 1989). Survivors of the original cohort were resurveyed in 1974 to obtain information on new morbidity and functional disability between 1965 and 1974. Data from both surveys also contain information on a large variety of behavioral and social risk factors that have been demonstrated to predict mortality (Wingard & Berkman, 1983). Further details of sampling methods and study design can be found in Berkman and Breslow (1983).

Mortality data reported in this chapter are based on the 2,424 men and 2,815 women in the Alameda County cohort who were aged 30 and over in 1965. There were a total of 676 deaths among men and 654 deaths among women between 1965 and 1983 resulting in crude mortality rates of 27.9% and 23.2% for men and women respectively. Data on self-reported new heart disease morbidity are based on the subset of those who did not report heart disease morbidity in 1965 and who responded to the resurvey in 1974. Cancer morbidity data are reported for those who did not have a previous diagnosis of cancer, and were obtained from population-based cancer incidence files (California Tumor Registry) maintained by the Cancer Prevention Section of the State of California Department of Health Services.

Figure 2.4 presents age-specific sex mortality ratios for cancer and heart disease in the Alameda County cohort for 1965 through 1983 (Wingard et al., 1989). There was a rapid decline in the heart disease sex mortality ratio with age which is consistent with the pattern noted in Figure 2.2 for United States vital statistics data for 1980. The sex mortality ratio for cancer shows a different age pattern than that for heart disease in the Alameda County Study. Note however, that the age pattern of the sex mortality ratio for cancer in the Alameda County Study cohort does differ from that found in U.S. vital statistics. The sex ratio for cancer mortality peaked between ages 60 through 69 in the Alameda County Study cohort and declined thereafter, while the sex mortality ratio for cancer peaked between ages 75 and 84 in the U.S. vital statistics data and did not show a marked decline after the peak. These data demonstrate an important difference (Morgenstern, Kleinbaum, & Kupper, 1980) between *rate* ratios based upon age-at-death (vital status data) and *risk* ratios which are based upon age-at-entry (cohort data). The longer the follow-up period, the greater the potential for classification differences between age-at-death and age-at-entry for each death that occurs. Conversely, when a particular birth cohort experiences an unusually large mortality risk due to an exposure at a single point in time (the "cohort effect"), age-at-event analysis may confuse cohort effects with age effects (Kleinbaum, Kupper, & Morgenstern, 1982). However, whether the age pattern for sex ratios based on rates and risks differ depends on the epidemiologic characteristics of the disease being investigated, as illustrated below for cancer mortality.

The difference between cancer mortality sex ratios by age-at-death (U.S. vital status data, Figure 2.2) compared to cancer mortality sex ratios by age-at-entry (Alameda County Study, Figure 2.4) may reflect two important epidemiologic characteristics of lung cancer mortality, which is the largest component of all cancer deaths for men. First, lung cancer appears to have a long latency period so that most lung cancer deaths occur after age 60 (age-at-event) (USDHHS, 1980). Secondly, sex ratios for lung cancer mortality reflect sex ratios for smoking exposure, which in turn depend on birth cohort membership (USDHHS, 1980). The large male excess in smoking exposure peaked in the 1930s among birth cohorts born about 1900 to 1910 (USDHHS,

Figure 2.4 Age-specific sex mortality ratio (M/F) for cancer and heart disease, Alameda County, CA, 1965 to 1983.

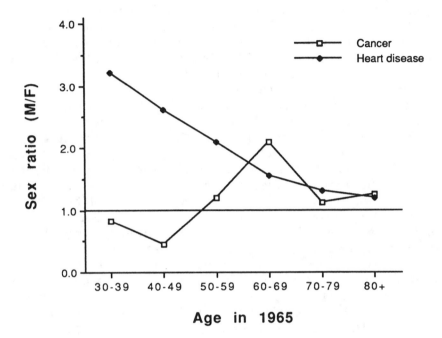

Age in 1965

Adapted from Wingard et al., 1989.

1980). Thus, the peak of the male excess in cancer mortality for those aged 60 through 69 at entry to the Alameda County Study in 1965 (birth cohorts 1896 to 1905) probably reflects the peak in male excess of cigarette smoking exposure for these birth cohorts (Cohn et al., 1987). Similarly, the high male excess for cancer death rates after age 70 observed in the U.S. vital status data in 1980 also reflects the experience of birth cohorts of males most heavily exposed to cigarette smoking who achieved ages 70 to 80 in 1980. Apparently, inconsistent age effects for the cancer mortality sex ratio when age-at-entry analyses are compared to age-at-event analyses can be explained by the epidemiology of cancer itself. Note that unlike results for cancer, rate and risk estimates of age effects for heart disease sex mortality ratios yield similar results, possibly reflecting the consistency of the sex mortality ratio for heart disease over time (Figure 2.1).

An in-depth analysis of sex ratios for health outcomes should also include a careful examination of sex specific effects (Wingard et al., 1989). For example, although the sex ratio (male/female) for both heart disease mortality and cancer mortality declines to near one in the oldest age groups in the Alameda County Study cohort (Figure 2.4), the path to that result is very different for these two outcomes. The convergence of male and female risk at older ages for heart disease mortality in the Alameda County Study cohort is due to an acceleration in female risk after ages 50 to 59 and a concomitant deceleration in male risk after ages 50 to 59 (Wingard et al., 1989). In contrast, the convergence of male and female risk for cancer mortality is due to a decline in risk among men after age 60 (Wingard et al., 1989). Female cancer mortality risk shows a fairly steady increase in risk from age 40. Thus, similar age patterns for sex ratios can be the result of very different sex-specific patterns.

Further variations in the sex ratio can be seen when morbidity and mortality are compared. Figure 2.5 presents sex ratios for heart disease morbidity and mortality for a nine-year follow-up of the Alameda County Study cohort (Wingard et al., 1989). (Note that differences between sex ratios for heart disease mortality given in Figures 2.4 and 2.5 reflect different lengths of follow-up for the two figures.) Figure 2.5 shows a large male excess of heart disease mortality for males at all ages, which contrasts with a female excess or male–female parity for heart disease morbidity. Others have noted that there is generally a female excess for mobidity, particularly for diseases that are not likely to be fatal (Hing et al., 1983; Verbrugge, 1980, 1985). In the Alameda County cohort we were able to confirm a female excess of morbidity even for heart disease, which is a leading cause of death in both men and women. Furthermore, a female excess for heart disease morbidity coexists with a male excess for heart disease mortality in the same population-based cohort.

The contradiction between sex ratios for heart disease morbidity and mortality is not consistent with results for cancer morbidity and mortality in the Alameda County cohort (Wingard et al., 1989). As can be seen in Figure 2.6, sex ratios for cancer morbidity and cancer mortality are very similar at all ages, and follow the same age pattern. Thus consistency of the sex ratio for morbidity and mortality depends on cause, and possibly on how morbidity is assessed. For example, sex differences in morbidity based on self-report may in part reflect sex differences in medical care utilization or reporting, while sex differences based on screening examinations will be less subject to these influences. Additionally, sex differences in morbidity based on prevalence rates (as opposed to incidence rates) will reflect both sex differences in incidence and survival.

Figure 2.5 Age-specific sex ratio (M/F) for heart disease morbidity and mortality, Alameda County, CA, 1965 to 1974.

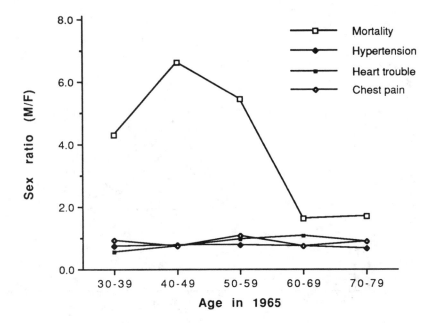

Adapted from Wingard et al., 1989.

SUMMARY

The major purpose of this chapter has been to illustrate that sex ratios for health demonstrate remarkable variability by age, cause, and type of endpoint (morbidity vs. mortality). These variations may provide important clues for understanding gender differences in health and longevity. Therefore, analytic tools, such as age-adjustment, which smooth these variations may obscure important clues. The use of the sex ratio itself may obscure important sex-specific patterns so that an examination of the numerator and denominator of the sex ratio may also provide important information. An examination of the variations in the sex differential by age, cause and outcome should lead to testable hypotheses concerning the biologic, behavioral, and psychosocial factors that result in the observed heterogeneity of the effect of gender on health.

Figure 2.6 Age-specific sex ratio (M/F) for cancer morbidity and mortality, Alameda County, CA, 1965 to 1983.

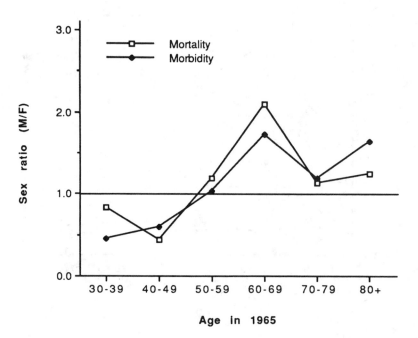

Adapted from Wingard et al., 1989.

ACKNOWLEDGMENT

This research was supported by the National Institute on Aging Grant #R01-AG05687 and #R29-AG08387.

REFERENCES

Berkman, L., & Breslow, L. (1983). *Health and ways of living: The Alameda County Study*. New York: Oxford Press.

Cohn, B. A., Wingard, D. L., Cirillo, P. M., Cohen, R. D., Reynolds, P., & Kaplan, G. A. (1987). Is cigarette smoking a stronger risk factor for lung cancer mortality for women than for men: prospective evidence from a cohort followed into the 1980s (abstract). *Am J Epidemiol, 126,* 767.

Hazzard, W. R. (1986). Biological basis of the sex differential in longevity. *J Am Ger Soc, 34,* 455–471.

Hing, E., Kovar, M. G., & Rice, D. P. (1983). Sex differences in health and use of medical care: United States. *Vital and Health Statistics,* Ser. 3, No. 24 Nat. Cent. Health Stat., DHHS Publ. (PHS):83-1408.

Johnson, A. (1977). Recent trends in sex mortality differentials in the United States. *J Hum Stress, 3,* 22–32.

Kleinbaum, D. G., Kupper, L. L., & Morgenstern, H. (1982). *Epidemiologic research: Principles and quantitative methods.* Belmont, CA: Lifetime Learning Publication.

Lopez, A. D. (1984). The sex differential in mortality in developed countries. In A. D. Lopez, & L. T. Ruzicka, (Eds). *Sex differentials in mortality: Trends, determinants and consequences,* (pp. 53–120). Canberra: Australian Nat. Univ. Press.

Morgenstern, H., Kleinbaum, D. G., & Kupper, L. L. (1980). Measures of disease incidence used in epidemiologic research. *International J Epidemiol, 9,* 97–104.

National Center for Health Statistics. (1983). Advance report, final mortality statistics, 1980. *Monthly Vital Stat Rep, 32,* (Suppl.).

National Center for Health Statistics. (1986). *Health, United States, 1986.* DHHS Pub. No. (PHS) 87-1232. Public Health Service: Washington, DC: U.S. Government Printing Office.

Preston, S. H. (1978). *Mortality pattern in national populations.* New York: Academic Press.

Retherford, R. D. (1975). *The changing sex differential in mortality.* Westport: Greenwood Press.

U.S. Department of Health and Human Services, Public Health Service, Office of the Assistant Secretary for Health, Office on Smoking and Health. (1980). *The health consequences of smoking for women: A report of the surgeon general.* Washington, DC: U.S. Government Printing Office.

Verbrugge, L. M. (1980). Recent trends in sex mortality differentials in the United States. *Women and Health, 5,* 17–37.

Verbrugge, L. M. (1985). Gender and health: An update on hypotheses and evidence. *J Health and Soc Beh, 26,* 156–182.

Waldron, I. (1974). Why do women live longer than men? *Soc Sci Med, 10,* 349–362.

Waldron, I. (1986). What do we know about causes of sex differences in mortality? A review of the literature. *Population Bulletin of the United Nations, 18,* 59–76.

Wingard, D. L. (1984). The sex differential in morbidity, mortality, and lifestyle. *Ann Rev Public Health, 5,* 433–458.

Wingard, D. L., & Berkman, L. (1983). A multivariate analysis of health practices and social networks. In L. Berkman & L. Breslow, (eds.) *Health and ways of living: The Alameda County Study.* New York: Oxford Press.

Wingard, D. L., Cohn, B. A., Kaplan, G. A., Cirillo, P. M., & Cohen, R. D. (1989). Sex differentials in morbidity and mortality risk examined by age and cause in the same cohort. *Am J Epidemiol, 130,*(3), 601–610.

II GENETIC AND BIOLOGIC BASES

3 Overview of Biomedical Perspectives: Possible Relationships between Genes on the Sex Chromosomes and Longevity

David W. E. Smith
Huber R. Warner

The striking differential in longevity that exists between men and women has been adequately documented in earlier chapters. While there is no doubt that social and behavioral factors play a major role in determining the average longevity of a population, or particular segments of a population, it is reasonable to speculate that biologic and genetic factors may also make some direct contributions to this "gender gap" in human society. This overview is intended to provide a rationale and perspective for considering biomedical aspects of the gender gap today, and to point out the questions that are discussed in more detail in the succeeding chapters by James Neel, Stanley Gartler, William Hazzard, and Marc Weksler. Because this and the following four chapters contain a large number of biological terms that may be unfamiliar to the nonbiologist reader, a glossary of these terms is provided at the end of this section.

The gender gap has developed and grown with the availability of modern standards of living, public health, and medical care; women have benefitted more than men. Human mortality increases with age and can usually be attributed to specific diseases or pathological processes. The leading causes of death have changed completely during this century from infectious diseases (tuberculosis was the most common cause of death in 1900) to ischemic heart disease, cancer, and cerebrovascular disease (Wingard, 1984). These changes in the diseases causing mortality occurred during the period when the gender gap grew from one or two years to seven or eight years in the United States, and when life expectancy at birth increased for each sex by about 50%. Thus, the gender gap is clearly accentuated as longevity increases, suggesting that factors involved in biological aging may also make important contributions to the gender gap. Therefore, the known biological differences between men and women must be considered for their possible contributions to the longevity differential.

THE GENOTYPE

The basis for this discussion is the well-known fact that while mammalian females have two X-chromosomes, males have a Y-chromosome and an X-chromosome. The X-chromosome of the male comes from the maternal gamete (ovum), and the Y-chromosome comes from the sperm. This means that one out of forty-six chromosomes differs extensively between human males and females. Whereas much progress has been made characterizing the X-chromosome, and in fact Victor McKusick refers to it as a pacesetter in human genetics research (McKusick, 1987), very little is known about the Y-chromosome.

The question of whether there is a female longevity advantage inherent in the female genotype compared to the male genotype, as was suggested by Montagu (1974), can be subdivided into several questions. The most important is, what are the genes on the X- and Y-chromosomes that might be critical to longevity (Smith & Warner, 1989)? The X-chromosome contains many genes involved in vital functions that are unrelated to female sex development (Sandberg, 1983). These include genes for molecules without which diseases such as hemophilia A, Duchenne muscular dystrophy (Koenig et al., 1987), Lesch-Nyhan syndrome (Stout & Caskey, 1985), and Hunter's syndrome (McKusick & Neufield, 1983) occur. The male is hemizygous for these genes, while in the female there are two alleles for each gene, and a single allele producing a functional gene product in the heterozygous female often results in a normal or viable phenotype.

Presumably, any essential function that maps on the X-chromosome, but whose function is not duplicated elsewhere, has the potential to confer greater longevity to the female. A few essential and conditionally essential genes are listed in Table 3.1. For example, the gene for a clotting factor may be considered to be conditionally essential because a defect in this gene is only important when bleeding occurs. Defects in blood clotting, immune functions, muscle function, and protection against oxidative damage may not be immediately lethal, but would certainly contribute to the longevity differential after birth. In contrast, any defect in nucleic acid biosynthesis is likely to lead to an aborted fetus and is less likely to contribute to the longevity differential after birth.

Table 3.1 Some Important Genes on the X-Chromosome

Gene	Gene Product	Cellular Role
HEMA	factor VIII (hemophilia)	Blood clotting
HEMB	factor IX (hemophilia)	Blood clotting
DMD/BMD	Dystrophin (muscular dystrophy)	Muscle function
G6PD	Glucose-6-phosphate dehydrogenase	Protection against ox- idative damage
?	DNA polymerase alpha	DNA synthesis
PRPS	Phosphoribosyl pyrophosphate syn- thetase	Nucleotide biosynthe- sis
HPRT	Hypoxanthine-guanine phospho- ribosyltransferase	Nucleotide biosynthe- sis
XLA	[a]	Immune response
XLA2	[a]	Immune response
SCIDX	[a]	Immune response

[a]Gene product is unknown.

Such a simple analysis is only part of the story, however. Men, while remaining apparently healthy for most of their lives, may eventually be at a disadvantage by virtue of having only one X-chromosome. While we can presume that most essential enzymes and other proteins are usually present in excess, there may also be rate-limiting processes which depend on expression of genes on the X-chromosome. During most of their lives, females do not express the genes on both of their X-chromosomes due to a process known as X-inactivation or Lyoniza-tion (Lyon, 1988). The inactivation of one X-chromosome in each cell early in female development, in order to achieve balanced gene dosage, would seem to negate some of the advantages of having two X chromo-somes (Gartler & Riggs, 1983; Lyon, 1972). After inactivation each female cell is functionally hemizygous, although the female mammali-an organism is a mosaic composed of both kinds of cells. In most mammals, inactivation is more or less random. Any explanation of a female longevity advantage based on the female genotope must consid-er the effects of X-chromosome inactivation.

There remains an advantage to the mosaic of functionally hemizygous cells in the case of heterozygotes for X-linked diseases in which biosynthetic defects in some cells can be compensated by neigh-boring cells with the other X-chromosome active. Gene products that have their effects extracellularly, such as blood clotting factor VIII (synthesized in the liver but active in the blood), and substances that can move from cell to cell need not be produced by every cell. Yet another mechanism occurs in muscle cells that are multinucleate. There is little, if anything, abnormal about the muscles and muscle function of the female heterozygote for Duchenne muscular dystrophy because of the representation of both kinds of nuclei in muscle cells (Walton, 1981).

There is also the possbility of cell selection during cell proliferation, depending on which X-chromosome is active. This occurs, for example, in heterozygotes with a deficiency in the enzyme hypoxanthine phosphoribosyltransferase (i.e., HPRT$^+$/HPRT$^-$) in which all red and white blood cells are of the kind that produce an active HPRT gene product. Selection seems to favor those stem cells of the hematopoietic system containing the intact gene for this purine scavanging enzyme, which has a predictable value in nucleic acid biosynthesis (Lyon, 1972; Stout & Caskey, 1985). One wonders how much plasticity there is in development following X-chromosome inactivation. Is it possible to develop an entire organ or perhaps an entire organism based on cell selection, from only those cells with one of the two X-chromosomes active that are able to proliferate and contribute to development?

Reactivation of genes on the X-chromosome may occur late in life as described in recent studies (Wareham, Lyon, Glenister, & Williams, 1987), and this phenomenon must be investigated to determine whether the process involves most or all of the genes on the inactive X-chromosome, and whether it occurs generally. If reactivation is a general phenomenon, its consequences must be investigated. It may be beneficial to females late in life by making needed genetic information available; on the other hand it may introduce deleterious gene imbalance late in life.

Much of the genetic content of the X-chromosome is presently unknown or is of uncertain significance to longevity, and the consequences of mutations of these genes have not been defined as sex-linked diseases. An example is the gene for the catalytic polypeptide of DNA polymerase α, the principal enzyme of eukaryotic DNA synthesis (Wang et al., 1985; Hanaoka, Tandai, Miyazawa, Hori, & Yamada, 1985), which also has been implicated in DNA repair (Tyrrell, Keyse, Amaudluz, & Pidoux, 1985). Cells lacking this enzyme activity would presumably be unable to proliferate. The X-linked gene for DNA polymerase α could function to a female advantage based on the proliferative ability of the cells of the female mosaic of hemizygous cells. Reactivation of the inactivated gene for the catalytic polypeptide late in life could provide an obvious survival advantage.

It is well recognized that the male-to-female ratio at conception is well over 1.0 (see Chapter 4, this volume). The ratio in abortuses is about 1.3, and it is reasonable that the ratio at conception is even higher. The ratio at birth is 1.05, indicating a substantial excess male mortality during the prenatal period. Some part of this early male die-off can be attributed to hemizygosity of the genes of the X-chromosome, and spontaneous abortuses commonly have chromosomal imbalances that often involve the sex chromosomes (Hassold, Quillen, & Yamane, 1983; McMillen, 1979). Does this early male die-off due to chromosomal imbalance and genetic disease continue to favor female longevity into later life?

The characteristics of the Y-chromosome are much in contrast to the X-chromosome. It is about a third the size of the X-chromosome, representing only 1.6% of the total chromosomal length. It is largely heterochromatic with DNA that is not expressed, and much of which is composed of repeated base sequences. It has significant areas of homology with the X-chromosome and with some of the autosomes. Among mammalian species there are large differences in the size of the Y-chromosome, and even among humans there is significant heterogeneity in the size of the chromosome, although there is little correlation between Y-chromosomal size and phenotypic characteristics (Sandberg, 1985). The variation and instability of the Y-chromosome are considered evidence of the genetic unimportance of most of the chromosome.

There are a few recognized genes that map to the Y-chromosome, with the most significant one being for a factor required for testicular differentiation. Page and colleagues (1987) extensively characterized a candidate gene and gene product for this function, but it has recently been questioned whether this gene or another mapping close to it is the critical gene for testicular differentiation (Burgoyne, 1989). The differentiation of the testis sets in motion the hormonal physiology of the mammalian male, while a second Y-chromosome gene appears to be necessary for spermatogenesis. These genes are located on the short arm of the Y-chromosome near the centromere. As will be discussed below and elsewhere in this volume, the male hormonal physiology affects longevity by several mechanisms.

Is there any genetic information on the Y-chromosome that could be a direct determinant of longevity, as opposed to determinants that operate through hormones? In mice, the Y-chromosome has a gene that interacts with autosomal genes in autoimmunity (Rosenberg & Steinberg, 1984). At the National Institutes of Health (NIH) Conference on Gender and Longevity, held in September 1987, Kirby D. Smith (Johns Hopkins) described an Amish family with a deletion in the distal part of the long arm of the Y-chromosome (Kunkel et al., 1977) that has a record of male longevity that exceeds that of American males, Amish males, and even American females. A recent paper from the Soviet Union (Kuznetsova, 1987) correlates more heterochromatin in the long arm of the Y-chromosome with male longevity. There are several possible interpretations of such findings, and it is not inconsistent that both deleted and added DNA could affect the expression of some determinant of longevity located on the long arm of the Y-chromosome. Because these changes do not involve the juxtacentromeric region of the Y-chromosome, where deletions are known to affect testicular differentiation, whatever effect there is on male longevity appears to be independent of sex hormones.

Also of some interest is the observation that the X-chromosomes inherited from males and females are different. In particular, the paternal X-chromosome is less methylated than the maternal X-chromosome (reviewed by Marx, 1988). This is not unexpected because X-chromosome inactivation is believed to be due in part to methylation of cytosine in DNA, and reactivation due to loss of such methyl groups (reviewed by Holliday, 1987; Lyon, 1988). Although there is no reason to suspect that this apparent methyl-directed imprinting of X-chromosomes contributes to the relative ability to express genes on the X-chromosomes in males and females, it does underscore the importance of understanding the relationship between methylation and gene expression in general.

A thorough understanding of the genetic factors discussed briefly above, and in more detail by Drs. Neel (Chapter 4) and Gartler (Chapter 5), will be necessary to appreciate the basis of the physiological differences discussed by Drs. Hazzard (Chapter 6) and Weksler (Chapter 7). The production of the appropriate sex hormones is obviously regulated by the X- and Y-chromosomes, but it is clear that these sex hormones also influence more than just sex determination. The effect of exogenous sex steroids on lipoprotein metabolism implies that endogenous steroids have comparable effects, even though the exact mechanisms of how these effects are mediated have yet to be elucidated.

SEX HORMONES

The modulation of the levels and the balance of the cholesterol-carrying lipoproteins by sex hormones is a major factor in the gender gap (see Chapter 6, this volume). As will be detailed there, sex hormones result in a healthier pattern of lipoproteins in women than men (Hazzard, 1986). The pattern in women undergoes a disadvantageous change at the menopause, and exogenous hormones, which are sometimes administered in the treatment of diseases, change the lipoproteins in patients in predictable ways. In the end, ischemic heart disease, consequent on atherosclerosis, is the principal cause of death of women, as it is of men, but the increased death rate with age from this disease lags behind that of men by several years, thus making a substantial contribution to the longevity differential.

Testosterone has effects on other systems and structures, for example the liver and the erythron (Bardin & Catterall, 1981), but it is difficult to relate these effects to a male disadvantage in longevity.

NEUROENDOCRINE EFFECTS, HORMONES, AND THE IMMUNE SYSTEM

Sex hormones and other hormones modulate longevity through their effects on behavior and through the immune system. These effects are interrelated, and the central nervous system is at the center of a complex relationship. Several points based on extensive research can be clearly stated in trying to sort out the complexities.

1. The brain is affected early in development by sex hormones that have several recognizable effects on central nervous system structure and function, although these are of unknown significance for longevity (MacLusky & Naftolin, 1981).

2. Sex hormones have well-recognized effects on the behavior of animals, with imprinting occurring during development and hormonal effects occurring throughout the life span, which affect such behavioral characteristics as aggressiveness, territoriality, mate selection, and mating behavior. Do these characteristics have their counterparts in humans leading to death through violence and other self-destructive behavior (Ehrhardt & Meyer-Bahlburg, 1981; Rubin, Reinisch, & Haskett, 1981)?

3. Abundant neuroendocrine connections exist by which the brain affects and is affected by hormonal secretions. Some, but not all, of these neuroendocrine connections operate through the hypothalamus and the anterior pituitary gland.

4. Reproductive senescence, which differs greatly as a process in males and females, makes a major contribution to aging phenotypes although it is not life-threatening and occurs well short of the life expectancy of humans and other mammals. Reproductive senescence includes cell depletion, cell death, and organ involution, and is subject to hormonal modulation (Finch, 1987; Vom Saal & Finch, 1988).

5. The central nervous system affects the immune system through neuroendocrine mechanisms that involve the hippocampus and which operate through glucocorticoids, which have well-known effects in reducing or moderating immune responses following stress (Munck, Guyre, & Holbrook, 1984). Sex hormones also affect the immune system (Grossman, 1985), with autoimmunity occurrng more commonly

in women and female rodents, and the progress of autoimmune diseases being slowed by castration and treatment with male hormones (Talal, 1981).

6. Behavior may have effects on the immune system. It is doubtful, for example, that all of the adverse effects of stress on the immune system are mediated through the adrenal cortex. An important question related to gender and longevity concerns the comparative effects of stress in the two sexes. Do the perception, handling, and physiological consequences of stress differ in men and women? What is the influence of age? As life-styles and roles change, these questions become ever more important (Sapolsky, Krey, & McEwen, et al., 1986).

While it is possible and, indeed, tempting to draw models with arrows connecting structures and processes to indicate relationships suggested by the above information, additional detailed and quantitative information must still be obtained by experiment and observation. Stress and violence are two phenomena with both biological and psychological aspects that can be investigated in humans and laboratory animals in the context of gender and longevity.

IMMUNE FUNCTION AND THE GENOTYPE

Most measures of immune function decline with age (Hausman & Weksler, 1985; see Chapter 7, this volume). It is assumed that the increased incidence with age of certain infectious diseases and neoplasms are a result of reduced immune competence. While there is some research suggesting a more rapid decline in immune function with age in men than in women (e.g., Mascart-Lemone, Delespesse, Servais, & Kunstler, 1982), much more work is needed, and, if the age-related decline is a basic difference of males and females, the mechanisms underlying the difference are important. The immune system in female mice does appear to be more robust than that in males, but it is not clear whether this has any direct relationship to the immunoglobulin genes that do map to the X-chromosome. There are, for example, several X-linked genes for B-lymphocyte function which are defective in cases of congenital immune deficiencies (Buckley, 1986). In one of these that causes agammaglobulinemia with some frequency, in heterozygous females there is cell selection in B-lymphocyte development, with the result that all B-lymphocytes have the nonmutant X-chromosome active (Fearon, Winklestein, Civin, Pardoll, & Vogelstein, 1987). While a female advantage in these diseases is most obvious in early postnatal life, it is possible that the female genotype has a role in stronger immune function in later life also.

QUESTIONS ABOUT THE LONGEVITY DIFFERENTIAL AS SEEN IN THE LATE 1980s

There are two questions that are interrelated, which cannot be answered with certainty today, and which concern the basic nature of the gender gap. These are:

1. How immutable is the human gender gap? It is of recent origin and it peaked in the U.S. at 7.8 years in 1970. It has decreased to 7.0 years during the 1980s because, while life expectancy has increased for both sexes, it has increased more for men. The death rate from ischemic heart disease has been declining for the past twenty years (Levy, 1981; Pell & Fayerweather, 1985) with the decline being greater in men, and with male longevity benefitting preferentially. Serum cholesterol and the manner of its handling and compartmentalization are significantly responsive to changes in diet, physical activity, smoking, and alcohol consumption. Death rates from ischemic heart disease even differ as to socioeconomic status (Hjermann, Holme, Byre, & Leren, 1981; Millar, 1983). Cholesterol-reducing drugs also have significant effects, and if their use becomes widespread much of the female advantage in coronary heart disease as modulated by sex hormones may disappear, and with it, much of the longevity differential (Angelin, Eriksson, & Einarsson, 1986; Illingworth, 1987). In postindustrial societies occupational and life-style factors contributing to mortality are changing, and while new problems may appear, some factors contributing in recognized ways to the gender gap are decreasing (e.g., Schoenborn, 1986).

2. Will there be a residual human gender gap after societal and cholesterol contributions are reduced or disappear? Are there other longevity determinants resulting from other male/female differences? What are these differences, and by what mechanisms do they result in a longevity advantage for women? Do they operate to reduce female vulnerability to the diseases of mortality? There are studies that show greater female survival to adult age in many animal species, both wild and domesticated (Hamilton, 1948), but these studies do not consider survival to an age approaching the species' life span (Smith, 1989). Wild animals die of predation and environmental causes, and even domesticated animals kept under carefully controlled conditions die of different causes than humans (Committee on Animal Models for Research on Aging, 1981). The gender gap seen in humans in our society in the late 1980s may be unique in that it is related to the diseases of human mortality at this time. Therefore, a failure to observe a female longevity differential in nonhuman mammals is not evidence that a female biological advantage may not exist in certain specialized settings.

The subsequent chapters in this section will detail what little we do know about the genetic and biologic basis of the longevity differential in 1990 and will focus our attention on the important questions that remain to be answered in this area. These include:

1. What genes on the X- and Y-chromosomes, if any, contribute directly to longevity?
2. How is the expression of these genes regulated?
3. Are there age-related differences in expression?
4. What biological functions other than sex determination are influenced by the sex hormones?
5. What role does the level of immune responsiveness play in health in late life?

REFERENCES

Angelin, B., Eriksson, M., & Einarsson, K. (1986). Combined treatment with cholestyramine and nicotinic acid in heterozygous familial hyper-cholesterolemia: Effects on biliary lipid composition *Eur. J. Clin. Invest. 16,* 391–396.

Bardin, C. W., & Catterall, J. F. (1981). Testosterone: A major determinant of extragenital sexual dimorphism. *Science 211,* 1285–1294.

Buckley, R. H. (1986). Humoral immunodeficiency. *Clinical Immunology and Immunopathology 40,* 13–24.

Burgoyne, P. S. (1989). Thumbs down for zinc finger? *Nature 342,* 860–862

Committee on Animal Models for Research on Aging (1981). *Mammaliam models for research on aging.* Washington, DC: National Academy Press.

Ehrhardt, A. A., & Meyer-Bahlburg, H. F. L. (1981). Effects of prenatal sex hormones on gender-related behavior. *Science 211,* 1312–1318.

Fearon, E. R., Winkelstein, J. A., Civin, C. I., Pardoll, D. M., & Vogelstein, B. (1987). Carrier detection in X-linked agammaglobulinemia by analysis of X-chromosome inactivation. *New England Journal of Medicine 316,* 427–431.

Finch, C. E. (1987). Neural and endocrine determinants of senescence: Investigation of causality and reproducibility by laboratory and clinical interventions. In H. R. Warner, R. N. Butler, R. L. Sprott, & E. L. Schneider (Eds.), *Modern biological theories of aging* (pp. 261–308). New York: Raven Press.

Gartler, S. M. & Riggs, A. D. (1983). Mammalian X-chromosome inactivation. *Annual Review of Genetics 17,* 155–190.

Grossman, C. J. (1985). Interactions between the gonadal steroids and the immune system. *Science 227,* 257–261.

Hamilton, J. B. (1948). The role of testicular secretions as indicated by the effects of castration in man and by studies of pathological conditions and the short lifespan associated with maleness. *Recent Progress in Hormone Research 3,* 257–322.

Hanaoka, F., Tandai, M., Miyazawa, H., Hori, T. & Yamada, M. (1985). Assignment of the gene for DNA polymerase alpha to the X chromosome. *Japanese Journal of Cancer Research (Gann) 76*, 441–444.

Hassold, T., Quillen, S. D., & Yamane, J. A. (1983). Sex ratio in spontaneous abortions. *Annals of Human Genetics 47*, 39–47.

Hazzard, W. R. (1986). Biological basis of the sex differential in longevity. *J. Am. Ger. Soc. 34*, 455–471.

Hausman, P. B., & Weksler, M. E. (1985). Changes in the immune response with age. In Finch, C. E., & Schneider, E. L., (Eds.), *Handbook of the biology of aging* (pp. 414–432). New York: Van Nostrand Reinhold.

Hjermann, I., Holme, I., Byre, K. V., & Leren, P. (1981). Effect of diet and smoking intervention on the incidence of coronary heart disease. *Lancet 2*, 1303–1310.

Holliday, R. (1987). X-chromosome reactivation. *Nature 327*, 661–662.

Illingworth, D. R. (1987). Long-term administration of lovastatin in the treatment of hypercholesterolaemia. *European Heart Journal 8*, Supplement E, 103–111.

Koenig, M., Hoffman, E. P., Bertelson, C. J., Monaco, A. P., Feener, C. & Kunkel, L. M. (1987). Complete cloning of the Duchenne muscular dystrophy (DMD) cDNA and preliminary genomic organization of the DMD gene in normal and affected individuals. *Cell 50*, 509–517.

Kunkel, L. M., Smith, K. D., Boyer, S. H., Borgaonkar, D. S., Wachtel, S. S., Miller, O. J., Breg, W. R., Jones, H. W. & Rary, J. M. (1977). Analysis of human Y-chromosome-specific reiterated DNA in chromosome variants. *Proc. Natl. Acad. Sci., U.S.A. 74*, 1245–1249.

Kuznetsova, S. M. (1987). Polymorphism of heterochromatin areas on chromosomes 1, 9, 16, and Y in long-lived subjects and persons of different ages in two regions of the Soviet Union. *Archives of Gerontology and Geriatrics 6*, 177–186.

Levy, R. I. (1981). Declining mortality in coronary heart disease. *Arteriosclerosis 1*, 312–325.

Lyon, M. F. (1972). X-chromosome inactivation and developmental patterns in mammals. *Biological Reviews 47*, 1–35.

Lyon, M. F. (1988). X-chromosome inactivation and the location and expression of X-linked genes. *Am. J. Hum. Gen. 42*, 8–16.

MacLusky, N. J., & Naftolin, F. (1981). Sexual differentiation in the central nervous system. *Science 211*, 1294–1303.

Marx, J. L. (1988). A parent's sex may affect gene expression. *Science, 239*, 352–353.

Mascart-Lemone, F., Delespesse, G., Servais, G., & Kunstler, M. (1982). Characterization of immunoregulatory T lymphocytes during ageing by monoclonal antibodies. *Clinical and Experimental Immunology 48*, 148–154.

McKusick, V. A. (1987). The morbid anatomy of the human genome: A review of gene mapping in clinical medicine. *Medicine, 66*, 237–296.

McKusick, V. A., & Neufeld, E. F. (1983). The mucopolysaccharide storage diseases. In J. B. Stanbury, J. D. Wyngaarden, D. S. Fredrickson, J. C.

Goldstein, & M. S. Brown (Eds.), *The Metabolic basis of inherited disease* (pp. 751–777). New York: McGraw-Hill.

McMillen, M. M. (1979). Differential mortality by sex in fetal and neonatal deaths. *Science 204,* 89–91.

Millar, W. J. (1983). Sex differentials in mortality by income level in urban Canada. *Can. J. Public Health 74,* 329–334.

Montagu, A. (1974). *The Natural superiority of women.* New York: Collier Books.

Munck, A., Guyre, P. M. & Holbrook, N. J. (1984). Physiological functions of glucocorticoids in stress and their relation to pharmacological actions. *Endocrine Reviews 5,* 25–44.

Page, D. C., Mosher, R., Simpson, E. M., Fisher, E. M. C., Mardon, G., Pollack, J., McGillivray, B., de la Chapelle, A. & Brown, L. G. (1987). The sex-determining region of the human Y chromosome encodes a finger protein. *Cell 51,* 1091–1104

Pell, S. & Fayerweather, W. E. (1985). Trends in the incidence of myocardial infarction and in associated mortality and morbidity in a large employed population, 1957–1983. *New England Journal of Medicine 312,* 1005–1011.

Rosenberg, Y. J., & Steinberg, A. D. (1984). Influence of Y and X chromosomes on B Cell responses in autoimmune prone mice. *J. Immunol. 132,* 1261–1264.

Rubin, R. T., Reinisch, J. M., & Haskett, R. F. (1981). Postnatal gonadal steroid effects on human behavior. *Science 211,* 1318–1324.

Sandberg, A. A. (Ed.) (1983). *Cytogenetics of the Mammalian X-Chromosome,* New York: Liss.

Sandberg, A. A. (Ed.) (1985). *The Y-Chromosome.* New York: Liss.

Sapolsky, R. M., Krey, L. C. & McEwen, B. S. (1986). The neuroendocrinology of stress and aging: The glucocorticoid cascade hypothesis. *Endocrine Reviews 7,* 284–301.

Schoenborn, C. A. (1986). Trends in smoking, alcohol consumption, and other health practices among U.S.A. adults, 1977 and 1983. *Advanced Data, National Center for Health Statistics,* 118.

Smith, D. W. E. (1989). Is greater female longevity a general finding among animals? *Biological Reviews 64,* 1–12

Smith, D. W. E. & Warner, H. R. (1989). Does genotypic sex have a direct effect on longevity? *Experimental Gerontology 24,* 277–288.

Stout, J. T., & Caskey, C. T. (1985). HPRT: Gene structure, expression, and mutation. *Annual Review of Genetics 19,* 127–148.

Talal, N. (1981). Sex steroid hormones and systemic lupus erythematosus. *Arthritis and Rheumatism 24,* 1054–1056.

Tyrrell, R. M., Keyse, S. M., Amaudruz, F., & Pidoux, M. (1985). Excision repair in U.V. (254nm) damaged non-dividing human skin fibroblasts: A major biological role for DNA polymerase alpha. *Int. J. Rad. Biol. 48,* 723–735.

Vom Saal, F. S., & Finch, C. E. (1988). Reproductive senescence: Phenomena and mechanisms in mammals and selected vertebrates. In E. Knobil (Ed.), *Physiology of Reproduction.* New York: Raven Press.

Walton, J. (Ed.) (1981). *Disorders of voluntary muscle*. Edinburgh: Churchill Livingstone.

Wang, T. S. F., Pearson, B. E., Suomalainen, H. A., Mohandas, T., Shapiro, L. J., Schroder, J. & Korn, D. (1985). Assignment of the gene for DNA polymerase alpha to the X chromosome. *Proc. Natl. Acad. Sci., U.S.A. 82,* 5270–5274.

Wareham, K. A., Lyon, M. F., Glenister, P. H. & Williams, E. D. (1987). Age related reactivation of an X-linked gene. *Nature 327,* 725–727.

Wingard, D. L. (1984). The sex differential in morbidity, mortality, and life-style. *Annual Review of Public Health 5,* 433–458.

GLOSSARY OF BIOLOGICAL TERMS

Alleles—Alternate states of individual genes that result in different phenotype, for example, blond vs. brown hair color.

Allogenic—Refers to genetically different members of the same species.

Androgen—A male steroid sex hormone

Aneuploidy—The state of containing an abnormal number of chromosomes.

Autosome—Any one of the nonsex chromosomes. They normally occur in pairs in all cells except sperm and egg cells.

Azacytidine—Analog of a normal constituent found in RNA and DNA. This compound inhibits methylation of these nucleic acids.

Centromere—The late-replicating region of a chromosome to which spindle fibers attach during cell division.

Concanavalin A—A plant protein that stimulates division of animal cells.

Congenic—Pertaining to strains that differ only in a single character or genetic region.

Demethylation—The process of removing methyl groups from nucleic acids.

Endoderm—The layer of cells lining the primitive gut in an embryo.

Epiblast—The outer germ layer of an embryo.

Epigenetic—A genetic change not due to mutation of the gene.

Estrogen—A female steroid sex hormone.

Gamete—A reproductive cell containing only one half the normal complement of chromosomes; a haploid germ cell.

Glucocorticoid—Steroid hormone produced by the adrenal gland.

Hemizygous—Pertaining to an individual who carries only one copy of a pair of genes, for example, found on the Y-chromosome.

Heterochromatic DNA—DNA containing highly repetitious sequences, and thought to be relatively inactive.

Heterogametic Sex—The sex that produces gametes containing unlike sex chromosomes, for example, male mammals that produce X- and Y-bearing sperm.

Heterosis—The greater vigor usually associated with hybrids or increased heterozygosity.

Heterozygous—A heterozygous individual carries a pair of different alleles of a particular gene.

Hippocampus—A region of the brain thought to be associated with memory.

Homozygous—Pertaining to an individual who carries a pair of identical alleles of a particular gene.

Hypertrophy—Excessive or uncontrolled growth of an organ or tissue.

Interphase—The phase during the cell cycle before the chromosomes begin to condense prior to cell division.

Involution—The process of decline or decay that occurs as an organism matures.

Karyotype—The chromosomal complement of an individual or species.

Lipopolysaccharide—A complex molecule composed of both lipid and polysaccharide components.

Lipoprotein—A complex molecule composed of both protein and lipid components.

Lymphocyte—An antibody-producing white blood cell.

Meiosis—The process of cell division to form germ cells in which each daughter cell carries one-half the usual number of chromosomes.

Methylation—The process of adding methyl groups to specific sites on DNA or RNA.

Monosomy—The condition resulting when a cell contains only one chromosome of a pair, instead of the usual two.

Oncogene—A gene involved in activating a cell to divide; uncontrolled expression of such a gene may lead to carcinogenesis.

Ontogeny—The development of an individual from an embryo to maturity.

Orchiectomy—Surgical removal of the testes.

Ovariectomy—Surgical removal of the ovary.

Parity—The state of having borne children.

Phagocytosis—The process of engulfing a cell or other large particle by another cell, such as a macrophage.

Phenotype—The observed characteristics resulting from a particular genetic background.

Phytohemagglutinin—A plant protein that stimulates animal cells to divide.

Syngeneic—Pertaining to genetically identical organisms.

Thymectomy—Surgical removal of the thymus.

Thymidine—A constituent of DNA.

Trisomy—The condition resulting when a cell contains an extra chromosome; thus, one kind of chromosome is present in triplicate.

4 Toward an Explanation of the Human Sex Ratio

James V. Neel

This chapter will consider in brief what we know about the puzzling departures of the sex ratios from unity. I use the plural because it is customary to recognize three sex ratios, namely, the primary sex ratio, established at conception; the secondary sex ratio, usually based on live- and stillbirths that have completed approximately seven months of gestation; and then what is termed the tertiary sex ratio, that which obtains at the age of reproduction.

THE SECONDARY SEX-RATIO

It is convenient to begin with a discussion of the secondary sex ratio, which is one of the most easily and accurately documented observations in human biology. Although there are occasional reports of populations with truly unusual sex ratios, in view of the amount of prenatal mortality we shall shortly consider and its potential impact on the sex ratio, the relative constancy in recent years of the secondary sex ratio, wherever in the world vital statistics are well reported, is impressive. In the United States, for example, the sex ratio for livebirths customarily reported as male births/female births $\times$ 100 is about 106 for livebirths to Caucasians and 103 for livebirths to blacks. The human male, as is true for mammalian males in general, is the heterogametic sex, and it has been generally assumed that the male produces X-bearing and Y-bearing sperm in equal numbers. Because the female is homogametic with respect to the X-chromosome, the expectation is for equal numbers of sexes at conception. Accordingly, ever since Painter elucidated the genetic basis for sex determination in humans in 1923, the observation of an excess of male births has piqued a wide variety of scientific interests.

Because the birth certificate usually records maternal age (and sometimes paternal age) and also maternal parity, there have been abundant data with which to search for age and parity effects on the sex ratio, as well, of course, as data to examine secular trends and the effect of certain sociological variables. An exhaustive review is not called for here, but the following papers provide examples of the data available. Among U.S. Caucasians, the sex ratio falls slightly with birth order and parental ages from, in the studies of Novitski and colleagues (1956, 1958), 106.6 among first born to 104.7 among eighth or later born. Interestingly, their analysis revealed that the factors in this fall were birth order and to a much lesser extent, *paternal* age; maternal age had no independent effect. A later analysis of another set of U.S. data by Erickson (1976) confirmed the birth order but not the paternal effect. The inference is that with successive births the uterus becomes relatively less hospitable to male fetuses, but however this is mediated, it is independent of an aging maternal physiology. Sex ratio has increased slightly in England and Scotland, and Wales since the turn of the century, but as Lowe and McKeown (1951) pointed out, stillbirths, with their relative excess of males, decreased during the same period; the inference is that improved living conditions, as reflected in a falling stillbirth rate, permit the livebirth of some males who would previously have been lost to stillbirths. Nothing fundamental has happened to the sex ratio.

THE PRIMARY SEX-RATIO

We turn now to a consideration of the primary sex ratio. For years it has been recognized that there is an excess of male births among abortuses, miscarriages, and still births, and efforts have been made to calculate a primary sex ratio on the basis of the observed sex ratio and the excess of males in abortions and miscarriages. These calculations have been severely hampered by poor data on total fetal loss and by difficulties in sexing early fetal losses on morphological grounds.

Two developments in the past several decades have now resulted in a much better estimate of this primary sex ratio, (a) carefully controlled studies on fetal loss in cohorts of women at risk of preganancy, and (b) sexing of early losses based on cytogenetic rather than morphological criteria. Longstanding scientific debate over the amount of so-called "fetal wastage" seems to have culminated in a consensus that at least 50% of conceptuses are lost, and the true figure may be as high as 60 or 70% (Abramson, 1973; Leridon, 1977; Roberts and Lowe, 1975). Preimplantation losses are difficult to evaluate, but in what appears to be the best study to date on postimplantation loss, it was 43% (Miller et al., 1980). I put the term "fetal wastage" in quotes because the word "wastage" has connotations of unnecessary and extravagant loss. As we will see, this is not actually the case.

The causes and implications of such high fetal losses are still being worked out. The classic picture taught in embryology courses of the human fetus peacefully floating in a water bed with nothing to do but eat and sleep is clearly incorrect. In terms of the struggle for survival, it is a jungle in there, prime time for natural selection.

The best evidence that a substantial portion of this total loss is selective comes from studies of the karyotypes of abortuses. Table 4.1 summarizes a great deal of work on this subject. Among early losses, more than 50% have gross chromosomal abnormalities. I use the term "gross" to designate abnormalities easily detected with light microscopy. Lesser chromosome abnormalities may of course be present in the apparently karyotypically normal. This demonstration of the amazingly high contribution of karyotypic abnormalities to early fetal loss in man is a major contribution of cytogenetics to our understanding of human biology.

There is also inferential evidence for fetal loss due to homozygosity for what we call point mutations, although this is much more difficult to document. A possible example stems from a survey of the frequency of heterozygous carriers of alleles associated with a battery of 12 enzyme deficiencies, conducted on infants live-born on the maternity service of the University of Michigan Hospitals. Among black infants, 4.8% were heterozygous carriers of a triosephosphate isomerase (TPI) allele associated with no enzyme activity (Mohrenweiser, 1983). TPI deficiency is generally recognized as the most severe of the glycolytic enzyme deficiencies and normally causes death before the age of 24 months. Based on the observed allele frequency of 0.024 in the black population, about one of every 2,000 newborn black infants would be expected to be homozygous for this allele, and yet to the date of that report (1983) only 18 homozygous deficient black infants had been recorded in the medical literature, in six families. This discrepancy may to some extent be due to failure to recognize this entity, but is more probably largely due to in utero death. Black infants comprised only 11.5% of the Ann Arbor series. On the basis of the more extensive data on Caucasians in that same series, we have estimated that at conception some 3% of Caucasoid conceptuses would have a near-total

Table 4.1 The Prevalence (per 1000) of Chromosome Anomalies in Spontaneous Abortions, Perinatal Deaths, and Livebirths[a]

Type of anomaly	Spontaneous abortions			Perinatal deaths (N = 500) (Machin, 1974)	Live-births (N = 43558) (Evans, 1977)
	< 12 weeks (N = 1498) (Boué et al, 1975)	< 18 weeks (N = 255) (Lauritsen, 1976)	< 28 weeks (N = 941) (Creasy et al, 1976)		
Tetraploidy	38.05	47.06	12.75	0	0
Triploidy	122.16	54.90	40.38	2.00	0.13
Autosomal trisomy	330.44	250.98	151.98	28.00	1.24
Monosomy X	93.46	156.86	72.26	2.00	0.046
Other	30.70	39.22	27.62	24.00	4.43
Total, all anomalies	614.81	549.02	304.99	56.00	6.26

[a]Adapted from J. Boué, A. Boué, & P. Lazar (1975). Retrospective and prospective epidemiological studies of 1500 karyotyped spontaneous human abortions. *Teratology, 12,* 11–26.

M. R. Creasy, J. R. Crolla, & E. D. Alberman (1976). A cytogenetic study of human spontaneous abortions using banding techniques. *Hum. Genet., 31,* 177–196.

H. J. Evans (1977). Chromosome anomalies among live births. *J. Med. Genet., 14,* 309–312.

J. G. Lauritsen (1976). Aetiology of spontaneous abortion. *Acta Obstet. Gynecol. Scand. (Suppl), 52,* 1–29.

G. A. Machin (1974). Chromosome abnormality and perinatal death. *Lancet, 1,* 549–551.

deficiency of some enzyme or the other (Mohrenweiser & Neel, 1981). It is reasonable to postulate that many of these infants would die in utero, as seems to be the case for the TPI-deficient black infants. Thus, the evidence now suggests that a high proportion of these early fetal losses occur for sound genetic reasons. The role in early fetal loss for maternal hormonal imbalance, morphological abnormality of the uterus, or malposition of the placenta—not to mention simple uterine capriciousness—is much less a factor than we thought only a few years ago.

As regards the sex ratio in these losses, the most accurate data should be derived from sexing on the basis of karyotype, that is, X- and Y-chromosomal constitution. Even here there is the possibility of error because of contamination of the fetal sample by maternal blood, Hassold and colleagues (1983) argued that this has introduced bias into many of the earlier karyotypic studies. Furthermore, with the demonstration that hydatidiform males are androgenetic in origin, these must be removed from any series concerned with the sex ratio in early fetal losses. Hassold et al. (1983) estimate that among karyotypically *normal,* spontaneously aborted fetuses, the sex ratio was approximately 130. The karyotypically *abnormal* spontaneously aborted fetuses must be divided into two groups, those characterized by abnormal numbers or combinations of sex chromosomes, among whom the designation of chromosomal sex may be considered moot, and those not so characterized, principally the autosomal trisomies. Among these latter the sex ratio was 115. Combining the data on sex ratio at birth with the data on the proportion of conceptuses lost and the sex ratio among them, Hassold et al. (1983) estimate that among conceptuses not characterized by sex chromosome aneuploidy, the sex ratio at conception is approximately 115.

The influence of parity on, and secular trends in, the sex ratio, as well as ethnic differences were mentioned earlier in this chapter. From the foregoing, it is clear that these are minor influences in comparison with the factors resulting in major change in the sex ratio between conception and term. Now that we are aware of how much in utero mortality there really is, most of these effects (lower sex ratio at advanced parity, lower sex ratio in American blacks, lower sex ratios in Great Britain at the turn of the last century) can be seen as the result of a response to more stringent intrauterine conditions. Given the "normal" amount of intrauterine mortality, it would require only a small tilt in the uterine environment to produce these changes.

Why this male preponderance in early losses, especially those with an apparently normal karyotype? An obvious and favorite speculation has been that this is due to the action of sex-linked alleles that are incompatible with survival in the hemizygous male. The mutations responsible for these alleles would either have just arisen in the mother or have been transmitted in the female line for several generations before finding expression in a male. Given our current understanding of the primary sex ratio, this suggestion will not withstand close scrutiny. If we assume an approximate genetic equilibrium with regard to the genes on the X-chromosome, we can infer an excess prenatal loss for genetic reasons of approximately 9% of male conceptuses from the difference between the primary and secondary sex ratio. We do not know how many loci capable of giving rise to prenatally lethal mutations are on the X-chromosome, but let us estimate about 1,000. This guesstimate is justified by the fact that the most current estimate of the number of "vital" genes in the mouse genome is 5,000–10,000 (Shedlovsky, Guenet, Johnson, & Dove, 1986) and humans are unlikely to have more than twice the genetic complexity of the mouse. Since the human X-chromosome is roughly 5% of the human (cytogenetic) genome, this leads to the figure of 1,000. To a first approximation, this implies a lethal mutation rate of almost 1×10^{-4}/locus/generation, which seems far too high. Another approach to the problem stems from the above-mentioned fact that the length of the X-chromosome is approximately 5% of the total genome. If the autosomes have the same rate of mutation to lethal genes as we have been forced to postulate for the X-chromosome, there should be roughly $(1.00 \times 0.09/0.05) = 1.8$ new *lethal* mutations in each gamete (not to mention other kinds of mutations). My arithmetic suggests that despite the high rate of in utero loss among karyotypically normal fetuses, the facts do not square with such a high total mutation rate, even if you make a generous allowance for provisional lethals and truncated selection. Unless you wish to believe that Mother Nature, for reasons known only to herself, engineered some kind of a death wish into the X-chromosome, it is difficult to argue that the differential prenatal loss of male fetuses can so simply be attributed to sex-linked mutations.

There is a factual as well as a theoretical basis for doubting that sex-linked mutations lethal in the male hemizygote in utero can be responsible for this heavy male mortality. From the recent studies on sex-linked Lesch-Nyhan syndrome, Duchenne's muscular dystrophy, chronic granulomatous disease, ichthyosis, and hemophilia A and B (Factor VIII and IX deficiency), it is known that even when hemizygous for a deletion, males may survive well into childhood (cf., Albertini, O'Neill, Nicklas, Heintz, & Kelleher, 1985; Ballabio et al., 1987; Kurachi & Chen, in press; Monaco, Bertelson, Colletti-Feener, & Kunkel, 1987; Royer-Pokora et al., 1986; Stout & Caskey, 1985; van

Ommen et al., 1985; Wilson et al., 1986; Yang et al., 1984; Youssoufian et al., 1987). One might expect that the presumably more extensive deletions that (as sex-linked lethals) result in male in utero deaths would also, because of Lyonization (see below), find some expression in females. This would result in pedigrees of apparent female-to-female transmission of a trait, the males being normal but the sex ratio being two females to one male. Unfortunately for this thought, Wettke-Schaffer and Kantner (1983) in a searching review of the literature (see also Happle, 1985) could find only three certain examples of this mode of inheritance (incontinentia pigmenti, oral-facial-digital syndrome I, and the focal dermal hypoplasia of Goltz). Among their possible additional examples for which the evidence is much weaker, even allowing for genetic heterogeneity in the syndrome, I can accept five (X-linked chondrodysplasia punctata, the Wildervanck syndrome, a form of congenital cataract with microcornea or slight microphthalmia, partial lipodystrophy with lipoatrophic diabetes and hyperlipidemia, and the Aicardi syndrome). For most of these latter examples, an autosomal dominant allele with lethality in males provides an equally good explanation. These entities are all quite rare. Their cumulative impact on the sex ratio, if this indeed is their mode of inheritance, would be quite small. It is difficult to believe there is a substantial number of such entities (minor manifestations in female heterozygotes, lethality in male hemizygotes) waiting to be discovered, and even more difficult to believe there is a considerable number of X-linked loci at which mutations resulting in early male death find no expression in female carriers. I do not mean to deny any role for sex-linked mutations in this excessive loss of males, but do feel it is not a sufficient explanation, in this respect endorsing the position adopted by Stevenson and Bobrow in their excellent review of 1967.

At this point I am moved to a small speculation. It is well known that inbreeding results in homozygosity, the children of first-cousin marriages being homozygous for alleles at 6% of their genetic loci; in our studies in Japan such liveborn infants exhibited a 17% increase in infant and juvenile mortality (Schull & Neel, 1965). A male even in the absence of inbreeding will be homozygous (more properly, hemizygous) for his genes in the X-chromosome (5% of his total genes). The female will be heterozygous for most of those alleles, albeit in the patchy fashion we associate with Lyonization (see below). One has to wonder whether despite Lyonization the female exhibits for X-linked genes a heterosis effect lacking in the male, an effect partially responsible for her greater survival.

Not only do we not, in my opinion, understand the reason for the excessive death of males in utero, we understand even less the reasons for the primary sex ratio. The standard surmise has been that the Y-chromosome bearing sperm, carrying less chromosomal baggage, can move faster. Recent studies analyzing human sperm chromosomes using zona-free hamster ova have made it clear that this is a rather demanding hypothesis—although none better is in sight. Kamiguchi and Mikamo (1986) report that in five studies, including their own, the ratio of X:Y sperm penetrating the hamster ova was 2543:2337, that is, 1.09 in favor of the X-chromosome bearing sperm. If for unknown reasons there really is a relative deficiency of Y-bearing (i.e., male-determining) sperm among mature spermatoza, this only enhances the mystery of the striking excess of males at the earliest stage of gestation at which the sex ratio has been determined.

The importance of the sex of the child being what it is in most cultures, interest in procedures to influence a prospective child's gender have a considerable and colorful history. Efforts to separate X- and Y-bearing sperm by various technical procedures go back at least 60 years (Lush, 1925) and have not been generally convincing (see references in Amann & Seidel, 1982; Erickson, Lewis, & Butley, 1981; Kaneko, Oshio, Kobayashi, Mohri, & Iizuka, 1984). Recently however, using discontinuous density gradient centrifugation of semen, Kaneko et al. (1984) have clearly demonstrated the production of a highly X-enriched fraction; Mohri and colleagues (1986) have presented limited clinical data demonstrating a significant excess of female offspring following the artificial insemination of women with this fraction. They conclude, in line with the suggestion of Erickson et al. (1981), that factors other than density differences are important in the separation of the two types of sperm. An obvious application of the technique is to increase the probability of female offspring in a family setting where the males are at increased risk of sex-linked disease. The possibility of more frivolous uses of the technique has sparked a lively discussion in Japan, where the technique was developed, concerning the ethics of use of the technique, a debate similar to that engendered earlier in the United States by the prospect of determining nuclear sex at an early fetal age in a society where most couples want at least one son and abortion is readily available. Given that the tertiary sex ratio is approximately unity (see below), any change in the secondary sex ratio—in either direction—would impact on the number of persons who in a monogamous society could not find mates.

THE TERTIARY SEX-RATIO

Males have long been known to exhibit a higher neonatal and child-hood mortality than females (reviewed in Scheinfeld, 1958). The result is that in recent years in most civilized countries, the sex ratio evens out about the third decade. However, the precise timing at which equality in the sex ratio is achieved is very much culture-driven. For instance, with the very low infant and child mortalities of the past several decades in the highly industrialized countries, the age at which the sexes become numerically equal is delayed.

Because this tertiary sex ratio is so culture-driven, it has less inherent biological interest than the primary and secondary sex ratios. However, there is a genetic component to the shift from a sex ratio of 106 to a ratio of 100 at age 30. This results from the lethal effects in childhood of such sex-linked genetic diseases as Duchenne's muscular dystrophy, hemophilia A, adrenoleukodystrophy, agammaglobulinemia, type VIII glycogen storage disease, chronic granulomatous disease, sex-linked hydrocephalus, Menke's syndrome, Hunter syndrome, and ornithine-transcarbamylase deficiency. The data do not permit an accurate estimate of the cumulative frequency with which these diseases will result in prereproductive death in males, but it is surely less than 1%. Thus, sex-linked disease in the strict sense can scarcely explain the excessive male mortality in the early decades of life.

Earlier the ability of genetic factors sensu strictu to explain the greater male mortality in utero was doubted. Now there is doubt that genetic factors can explain the greater male mortality which usually obtains between birth and maturity, that is, that primary genetic mechanisms account for all the excess male mortality in early life. This shifts much of the burden of responsibility to the fact of maleness itself. To be sure, this is genetically determined, but however "maleness" works, I would term it a secondary or derivative genetic mechanism. Thus, males cannot take refuge in their extra load of sex-linked mutations as an explanation of their higher death rates from conception to adulthood, but must entertain the possibility that they really are the weaker sex as judged by survival, biologically less fit than females from the outset.

There is still one avenue by which genetics could play a role in the reduced survival of males not attributable to sex-linked genes. Genetic theory holds that all of us carry in the heterozygous state a number of deleterious autosomal genes, which if rendered homozygous would handicap our functioning in some way. Inbreeding, as mentioned earlier, results in increased homozygosity for these genes. One might surmise that this increased mortality would fall more heavily on the male sex if the male is in some undefined way the weaker. Only one major study has examined this possibility. Schull (1958), in the extensive data set on the outcome of consanguineous marriages assembled in connection with studies of the genetic effects of the atomic bombs (see below), found no change in the sex ratio in relation to inbreeding. Thus, we have no hard evidence for genetic effects other than those mediated through sex-linkage in the excess male mortality.

RADIATION AND THE SEX RATIO

In closing I turn briefly to my principal personal involvement with the study of sex ratio. When organizing the studies on the potential genetic effects of the atomic bombs in Hiroshima and Nagasaki in 1946–1947 (cf., Neel & Schull, 1956), I felt that alterations in the sex ratio would be one legitimate indicator of such an effect. The argument was very simple—too simple, as it turned out. The male receives his single X-chromosome from his mother, whereas the female receives one X from her mother and the other from her father. In the event of maternal radiation, the hemizygous males should experience the consequences of both sex-linked recessive and dominant deleterious mutations operating prenatally, whereas the female should exhibit only the consequences of dominant mutation. Because recessive mutations are more common than dominant, the net effect of maternal radiation was expected to be a depression of the sex ratio. In the event of paternal radiation, since the male transmits his X to his daughters only, any deleterious mutations impairing prenatal survival should result in an increase in the sex ratio.

Data on the sex ratio were collected for some 20 years following the bombings. During that period, human cytogenetics came of age, and two potential complications in the interpretation of any sex ratio changes in these children became apparent. The first was the phenomenon of Lyonization of one of the X-chromosomes in females, as described by Dr. Gartler (Chapter 5, this volume). This means that a female heterozygous for a sex-linked allele lethal in males is a mosaic of normal and abnormal tissue, and just how these two sets of tissue interact is not yet clear. Thus, in the event of paternal radiation, it could not be anticipated what proportion, if any, of the induced mutations would be expected to find expression in the daughters of exposed males. The second complication was the recognition of sex chromosome aneuploids, individuals who as a consequence of nondisjunction of the sex chromosomes at meiosis had abnormal complements of the sex chromosomes, such as XO, XXY, XXX, and XYY. Chromosomal nondisjunction was the first demonstrated genetic effect of radiation, by Mavor in 1921 in experiments with Drosophila, although to be sure at monstrous doses compared with the situation in Japan. Because the

relative proneness of men and women to this potential effect of radiation was unknown, and since the survival of these various types of
aneuploids appears to be unequal, XO types having a relatively high in
utero mortality, there was no a priori basis for an expectation, and so
no way to make allowance for this phenomenon in interpreting any
findings regarding sex ratio. These developments forced us to set aside
the study of sex ratio in this context for awhile.

Fortunately for our efforts to use sex ratio to study the genetic effects
of the atomic bombs, Awa and his colleagues during the past 20 years
have mounted an extensive cytogenetic study of the offspring of survivors and a suitable control group (Awa et al., 1987). Their subjects
were in part a subset of the larger sample in which we studied sex
ratio. The findings with respect to the sex-chromosome aneuploids are
given in Table 4.2. There is no obvious effect of parental exposure on
the frequency of sex-chromosomal aneuploids.

With the assurance that an increase in sex-chromosome aneuploids
is not distorting the sex ratio in these children, we have now returned
to this subject, reconsidering the results of an analysis conducted in
1966 (Schull, Neel, & Hashizume, 1966). However, because of the
uncertainty that Lyonization introduces regarding the survival of
females carrying alleles lethal in the male, we will be concerned only
with the results of maternal radiation. Regardless of how Lyonization
influences the expression of sex-linked lethal genes, the expectation is
that if sex-linked mutations were induced in the mother a greater
decrease in males than females would occur, that is, a negative regression of proportion of male births on maternal exposure. In fact, in the
clearest set of data, where only the mother was exposed, the regression
term was positive, albeit insignificantly so (0.0027/Sv). The average
maternal gonad exposure in this series of mothers is estimated to be
approximately 0.24 Sv, with individual gonad exposures ranging from
0.01 Sv to 2.50 Sv.

Thus, the sex ratio provides no evidence for a genetic effect of the
atomic bombs. By the standards of the radiation geneticist, however,
the gonad exposures experienced by these mothers were relatively
small. By itself, this one observation is certainly inadequate to evaluate the genetic effects of the atomic bombs. However, a variety of
other endpoints (congenital defects/stillbirths, survival of liveborn infants, sex-chromosome aneuploids, balanced reciprocal chromosomal
translocations, protein abnormalities detectable by electrophoresis,
and malignancies in the children of survivors) are also showing little
or no difference in frequency in the children of exposed and of nonex-
posed parents. We are beginning to develop the case for humans being
rather less sensitive to the genetic effects of radiation than had been

Table 4.2 The Prevalence (per 1000) of Children Found to Have Sex Chromosome Abnormalities among the Offspring of Survivors of the Atomic Bombings and a Suitable Comparison Population[a]

	Males					Females				
	XYY	XXY	Mosaic	Other	Total	X	XXX	Mosaic	Other	Total
Hiroshima										
Control	5(2.02)	4(1.61)	0	2(0.81)	11(4.44)	0	3(1.14)	3(1.14)	0	6(2.28)
Exposed										
Father	0	1(1.57)	1(1.57)	0	2(3.13)	0	2(3.14)	0	0	2(3.14)
Mother	0	4(2.97)	0	0	4(2.97)	0	1(0.67)	0	0	1(0.67)
Both	0	1(3.65)	0	0	1(3.65)	0	1(3.03)	1(3.03)	0	2(6.06)
Total	0	6(2.65)	1(0.44)	0	7(3.10)	0	4(1.63)	1(0.41)	0	5(2.04)
Nagasaki										
Control	0	5(4.15)	0	0	5(4.15)	0	1(0.60)	0	1(0.60)	2(1.21)
Exposed										
Father	2(3.68)	0	0	0	2(3.68)	0	1(1.61)	0	0	1(1.61)
Mother	1(1.10)	1(1.10)	0	1(1.10)	3(3.29)	0	0	1(0.89)	0	1(0.89)
Both	0	0	0	0	0	0	0	0	0	0
Total	3(1.81)	1(0.60)	0	1(0.60)	5(3.02)	0	1(0.51)	1(0.51)	0	2(1.02)
Total										
Control	5(1.36)	9(2.44)	0	2(0.54)	16(4.35)	0	4(0.93)	3(0.70)	1(0.23)	8(1.86)
Exposed										
Father	2(1.69)	1(0.85)	1(0.85)	0	4(3.39)	0	3(2.38)	0	0	3(2.38)
Mother	1(0.44)	5(2.11)	0	1(0.44)	7(3.10)	0	1(0.38)	1(0.38)	0	2(0.77)
Both	0	1(2.11)	0	0	1(2.11)	0	1(1.87)	1(1.87)	0	2(3.73)
Total	3(0.77)	7(1.79)	1(0.26)	1(0.26)	12(3.07)	0	5(1.13)	2(0.45)	0	7(1.59)
Newborn infants[b]	35(0.93)	35(0.93)	14(0.37)	14(0.37)	98(2.59)	2(0.10)	20(1.04)	7(0.37)	0	20(1.51)
No. of cases					37,779					19,173

The rates for the sex chromosome abnormalities apply only to the affected sex.

[a]Data from Awa et al. (1987).

[b]Cited from Hook and Hamerton (1977).

projected from studies on mice, up to now the chief human surrogate in the field of genetics for developing legislation and regulation regarding radiation exposures (Schull, Otake, & Neel, 1981; Neel, in press).

SUMMARY

The ratio at conception of males to females has been estimated to be about 115. Because the sex ratio at birth is usually between 103 and 106, it is clear that there is excessive male mortality in utero. Because this mortality can be only partially accounted for by sex-linked alleles in the hemizygous male, it appears that maleness per se is associated with higher mortality rates than femaleness. However, the reason for this higher male morality rate remains elusive. Equally elusive is the explanation for the high sex ratio at conception, as there is no evidence that Y-chromosome bearing sperm are more capable of penetrating ova than are X-chromosome bearing sperm. Finally, it also remains to be determined whether the excessive male mortality in utero is due to the same causes as it is after birth, as the sex ratio continues to fall after birth, on a variable schedule depending on the harshness of the environment. These questions will provide major challenges for research on the gender gap in the 1990s.

REFERENCES

Abramson, F. D. (1973.) Spontaneous fetal death in man. *Social Biology, 20,* 375–403.

Albertini, R. J., O'Neill, J. P., Nicklas, J. A., Heintz, N. H., & Kelleher, P. C. (1985). Alterations of the *hprt* gene in human *in vivo*-derived 6-thioguanine-resistant T lymphocytes. *Nature, 316,* 369–371.

Amann, R. P., & Seidel, G. E., Jr. (1982). *Prospects for sexing mammalian sperm.* Boulder: Colorado Associated University Press.

Awa, A. A., Honda, T., Neriishi, S., Sofuni, T., Shimba, H., Ohtaki, K., Nakano, M., Kodama, Y., Ito, M., & Hamilton, H. B. (1987). Cytogenetic studies of the offspring of atomic bomb survivors. In G. Obe & A. Basler (Eds.), *Cytogenetics: Basic and Applied Aspects.* Berlin: Springer-Verlag. pp. 166–183.

Ballabio, A., Parenti, G., Carrozzo, R., Sebastio, G., Andria, G., Buckle, V., Fraser, N., Craig, I., Rochi, M., Romeo, G., Jobsis, A. C., & Persico, M. G. (1987). Isolation and characterization of a steroid sulfatase cDNA clone: Genomic deletions in patients with X-chromosome-linked ichthyosis. *Proceedings of the National Academy of Sciences USA, 84,* 4519–4529.

Erickson, J. D. (1976). The secondary sex ratio in the United States 1969–

1971: Association with race, parental ages, birth order, paternal education and legitimacy. *Annals of Human Genetics, 40,* 205–212.

Erickson, R. P., Lewis, S. E., & Butley, M. (1981). Is haploid gene expression possible for sperm antigens? *Journal of Reproductive Immunology, 3,* 195–217.

Evans, H. J. (1984). Genetic damage and cancer. In J. M. Bishop, J. D. Rowley, & M. Greaves (Eds.), *Genes and Cancer.* New York: Liss.

Happle, R. (1985). Lyonization and the lines of Blaschko. *Human Genetics, 7,* 200–206.

Hassold, T., Quillen, S. D., & Yamane, J. A. (1983). Sex ratio in spontaneous abortions. *Annals of Human Genetics, 47,* 39–47.

Hook, E. B., & Hammerton, J. L. (1977). The frequency of chromosome abnormalities detected in consecutive newborn studies—differences between studies—results by sex and by severity of phenotypic involvement. In E. B. Hook & I. H. Proter (Eds.), *Population cytogenetics* (pp. 63–79). New York: Academic Press.

Kamiguchi, Y., & Mikamo, K. (1986). An improved, efficient method for analyzing human sperm chromosomes using zona-free hamster ova. *American Journal of Human Genetics, 38,* 724–740.

Kaneko, S., Oshio, S., Kobayashi, T., Mohri, H., & Iizuka, R. (1984). Selective isolation of human X-bearing sperm by differential velocity sedimentation in Percoll density gradients. *Biomedical Research, 5,* 187–194.

Kurachi, K., & Chen, S. H. (in press). Molecular genetic analysis of congenital disease: Human factor IX disorders. In M. M. Bern & F. Frigoletto (Eds.), *Hematologic contributions to fetal health.* New York: Liss.

Leridon, H. (1977). *Human fertility.* Chicago: University of Chicago Press.

Lush, J. L. (1925). The possibility of sex control by artificial insemination with centrifuged spermatozoa. *Journal of Agricultural Research, 30,* 893–913.

Lowe, C. R., & McKeown, T. (1951). A note on secular changes in the human sex ratio at birth. *British Journal of Social Medicine, 5,* 91–97.

Mavor, J. W. (1921). On the elimination of the x-chromosome from the egg of *Drosophila melanogaster* by x-rays. *Science, 54,* 277–279.

Miller, J. F., Williamson, E., Glue, J., Gordon, Y. B., Grudzinskas, J. G., & Skyes, A. (1980). Fetal loss after implantation. *Lancet, 2,* 554–556.

Mohrenweiser, H. W. (1983). Enzyme-deficiency variants: Frequency and potential significance in human populations. In M. C. Rattazzi, J. G. Scandalios & G. S. Whitt (Eds.), *Isozymes: Current Topics in Biological and Medical Research, Vol. 10: Genetics and Evolution* (pp. 51–68). New York: Liss.

Mohrenweiser, H. W., & Neel, J. V. (1981). Frequency of thermostability variants: Estimation of total "rare" variant frequency in human populations. *Proceedings of the National Academy of Sciences USA, 78,* 5729–5733.

Mohri, H., Oshio, S., Kaneko, S., Kobayashi, T., & Iizuka, R. (1986). Separation and characterization of mammalian X- and Y-bearing sperm. *Development, Growth, & Differentiation, 28,* 35–36.

Monaco, A. P., Bertelson, C. J., Colletti-Feener, C. & Kunkel, L. M. (1987). Localization and cloning of Xp21 deletion breakpoints involved in muscular dystrophy. *Human Genetics, 75,* 221–227.

Neel, J. V. (in press). Reproductive and genetic effects of gonadal exposure to ionizing radiation in human beings. In J. Mulvihill & R. J. Sherins (Eds.), *International Conference on Reproduction and Human Cancer.* New York: Raven Press.

Neel, J. V., & Schull, W. J. (1956). The Effect of Exposure to the Atomic Bombs, on Pregnancy Termination in Hiroshima and Nagasaki. *National Academy of Sciences-National Research Council,* Publ. 461.

Novitski, E., & Sandler, L. (1956). The relationship between parental age, birth order and the secondary sex ratio in humans. *Annals of Human Genetics, 21,* 123–131.

Novitski, E., & Kimball, A. W. (1958). Birth order, parental ages, and sex of offspring. *American Journal of Human Genetics, 10,* 268–275.

Painter, T. S. (1923). Studies in mammalian spermatogenesis II. The spermatogenesis of man. *Journal of Experimental Zoology,* 37: 291–334.

Roberts, C. J., & Lowe, C. R. (1975). Where have all the conceptions gone? *Lancet, 1,* 498–499.

Royer-Pokora, B., Kunkel, L. M., Monaco, A. P., Gott, S. C., Newburger, P. E., Baehner, R. L., Cole, F. S., Curnutte, J. T., & Orkin, S. H. (1986). Cloning the gene for the inherited disorder chronic granulomatous disease on the basis of its chromosomal location. In *Molecular Biology of* Homo sapiens, *Cold Spring Harbor Symposium on Quantitative Biology, Vol. LI,* Cold Spring Harbor Laboratory, Cold Spring Harbor, N. Y.

Scheinfeld, A. (1958). The mortality of men and women. *Scientific American, 198,* 22–27.

Schull, W. J. (1958). Empirical risks in consanguineous marriages: sex ratio, malformation, and viability. *American Journal of Human Genetics, 10,* 294–343.

Schull, W. J., & Neel, J. V. (1965). *The effects of inbreeding on Japanese children.* New York: Harper & Row.

Schull, W. J., Neel, J. V., & Hashizumi, A. (1966). Some further observations on the sex ratio among infants born to survivors of the atomic bombings of Hiroshima and Nagasaki. *American Journal of Human Genetics, 18,* 328–338.

Schull, W. J., Otake, M., & Neel, J. V. (1981). Hiroshima and Nagasaki: A reassessment of the mutagenic effect of exposure to ionizing radiation. In E. B. Hook & I. H. Porter (Eds.), *Population and Biological Aspects of Human Mutation.* New York: Academic Press.

Shedlovsky, A., Guenet, J. L., Johnson, L. L., & Dove, W. F. (1986). Induction of recessive lethal mutations in the T/t-H-2 region of the mouse genome by a point mutagen. *Genetical Research, 47,* 135–142.

Stevenson, A. C., & Bobrow, M. (1967). Determinants of sex proportions in man, with consideration of the evidence concerning a contribution from X-linked mutations to intrauterine death. *Journal of Medical Genetics, 4,* 190–221.

Stout, J. T., & Caskey, C. T. (1985). HPRT: Gene structure, expression and mutation. *Annual Review of Genetics, 19,* 127–148.

van Ommen, G. J. B., Verkerk, J. M. H., Hofker, M. H., Monaco, A. P., Kunkel, L. M., Ray, P., Worton, R., Wieringa, B., Bakker, E., & Pearson, P. L. (1986). A physical map of 4 million bp around the Duchenne Muscular Dystrophy gene on the human x-chromosome. *Cell, 47,* 499–504.

Wettke-Schafer, R., & Kantner, G. (1983). X-linked dominant inherited diseases with lethality in hemizygous males. *Human Genetics, 64,* 1–23.

Wilson, J. M., Stout, J. T., Palella, T. D., Davidson, B. L., Kelley, W. N., & Caskey, C. T. (1986). A molecular survey of hypoxanthine-guanine phosphorbosyltransferase deficiency in man. *Journal of Clinical Investigation, 77,* 188–195.

Yang, T. P., Patel, P. I., Chinault, A. C., Stout, J. T., Jackson, L. G., Hildebrand, B. M., & Caskey, C. T. (1984). Molecular evidence for new mutation at the *hprt* locus in Lesch-Nyhan patients. *Nature, 310,* 412–414.

Youssoufian, H., Antonarakis, S., Aronis, S., Tsoftis, G., Phillips, D., & Kazazian, H. H. (1987). Characterization of five partial deletions of the factor VIII gene. *Proceedings of the National Academy of Sciences USA, 84,* 3773–3776.

5 The Relevance of X-Chromosome Inactivation to Gender Differentials in Longevity

Stanley M. Gartler

INTRODUCTION

In this chapter the possible relevance of X-chromosome inactivation to the gender difference in longevity is considered. The basic cell and molecular biology of X inactivation is reviewed and three aspects of the X-inactivation process that may affect the sexes in a differential manner are discussed. The embryology of X inactivation is looked at as a developmental load unique to the female and, consequently, one in which error will primarily affect the female. Such errors could contribute to the well-known sex ratio of more males than females found in essentially all populations. The maintenance of X inactivation requires some degree of renewal at every cell division and again is largely a load unique to the female. However, it is not clear how errors in maintenance will affect the gender gap difference. Finally, the mosaic nature of the female resulting from X inactivation is discussed. Mosaicism makes possible cell selection, and several instances of adaptive cell selection are pointed out and their relevance to the gender gap in longevity is considered.

GENETIC BIOLOGY OF X INACTIVATION

In species with XY systems of sex determination, such as in humans, the expression of the two X chromosomes in the female is generally equivalent to the one X in the male in somatic cells. This phenomenon, which has been studied since the 1930s when it was first described in fruit flies is called dosage compensation (Muller, League, & Offerman, 1931). The particular form which it takes in most mammals, including humans, is called X-chromosome inactivation (Lyon, 1961). As the name implies, dosage compensation is achieved by inactivating one of the two X chromosomes in the female, thereby making the two Xs in the female equivalent to the one X in the male. The ontogeny of mammalian dosage compensation is fairly complex and seems to follow a series of early developmental cues. X inactivation first occurs in the trophectoderm where it is nonrandom, with the paternal X chromosome being preferentially inactivated. It takes place next in the primitive endoderm, which is another extra-embryonic derivative like the trophectoderm, and again inactivation is nonrandom with the paternal X chromosome being preferentially inactivated (Gartler & Riggs, 1983).

When the epiblast, which is the source of the embryo proper, differentiates, inactivation occurs again, but this time it is random with either the paternal or maternal X being inactivated. Once inactivation takes place in a cell, whether it is the maternal or paternal X, that pattern of inactivation becomes a fixed part of the cell's somatic heredity. The female becomes a mosaic with some cell lines expressing the maternal X chromosome and other cell lines expressing the paternal X. Presumably, all the cells in the epiblast are subject to inactivation including germ line stem cells. However, when the female germ line enters meiosis, reactivation of the inactive X occurs, and so throughout oogenesis the oocyte contains two active X chromosomes. In the male with one X chromosome there is, of course, no inactivation in somatic cells; however, in spermatogenesis the single X chromosome undergoes a precocious condensation and inactivation that appears critical to fertility in the male (Gartler & Riggs, 1983).

MOLECULAR BIOLOGY OF X INACTIVATION

In interphase cells the inactive X chromosome forms a heterochromatic structure called sex chromatin and like other forms of heterochromatin it is transcriptionally inactive and late replicating. At the cytological level it appeared that the entire X chromosome was inactivated. However, it has recently been shown that a true XY pairing region exists in mammals, and genes in the region have functional alleles on both the X and Y chromosomes, and as expected escape X inactivation (Keitges, Schorderet, & Gartler, 1987; Rouyer et al., 1986).

At the molecular level we now have evidence from studies of several X-linked housekeeping genes that the 5' ends of these genes are distinguished by methylation and nuclease sensitivity differences. The genes on the inactive X are hypermethylated relative to the alleles on the active X. That these differences are functional is supported by the fact that inactive X-linked genes can be reactivated by the powerful demethylating agent 5-azacytidine (5AC), and then shown to have become both demethylated at their 5' ends and nuclease sensitive (Riggs, Singer-Sam, & Keith, 1985; Riley, Goldman, & Gartler, 1986; Toniolo, Martini, Migeon, & Dono, 1988; Wolf, Jolly, Lunnen, Friedmann, & Migeon, 1984). Though the methylation differences between active and inactive X-linked alleles are functional, they are most likely not primary. A simplified model of X inactivation has been proposed in which the initial event is sex chromatin formation unaccompanied by methylation differences of individual loci (Gartler, Dyer, Graves, & Rocchi, 1985; Kratzer, Chapman, Lambert, & Evans 1983; Lock, Takagi, & Martin, 1987). In extra-embryonic cells where X inactivation begins, sex chromatin would be the only level of repression of genes on the inactive X. When inactivation occurs in the embryo proper, sex chromatin formation is again the initial event but is followed by differential methylation as part of a fail safe or locking device. Thus, the inactive X in somatic cells in transcriptionally repressed by both heterochromatinization in the form of sex chromatin and hypermethylation.

The focus of this chapter is to consider what contribution, if any, X inactivation might make to the gender gap in longevity. There are a number of ways in which X inactivation might affect females and males in a differential way and possibly contribute to the difference in life expectancy of males and females; these will be considered in the following order: the effect on the female of the embryology of X inactivation, errors in the maintenance of the X-inactivation system, and the mosaic nature of the female and somatic cell selection.

POSSIBLE EFFECTS OF THE EMBRYOLOGY OF X INACTIVATION ON THE GENDER GAP IN AGING

The embryology of X inactivation involves a complex set of events, and errors in any one of them will have serious consequences. Initiation of X inactivation most likely depends on an intracellular assessment of the X:autosome ratio. A ratio of 1:2 as found in male cells should exclude inactivation while a ratio of 1:1 as found in female cells should signal initiation. Errors at this point, that is, inactivation in a male cell, would certainly result in cell lethality and failure of X inactivation in a female embryo should create an aneuploidy effect. The fact that no female embryo or fetus has been observed without X inactivation supports this notion and implies that such an aneuploidy effect might lead to early embryonic lethality.

Once X inactivation is initiated in the female embryo, sex chromatin must form, a process that may involve a number of steps. It should be paternal in the extra-embryonic lineages and then random in embryonic cells. Differential methylation must follow, and errors in any one of those steps should lead to an apparently serious aneuploidy effect in the female. Another critical embryological event involving X inactivation in the female is reactivation in the germ line, which occurs at the entry to meiosis. Failure of this step should not produce an aneuploidy effect but would probably lead to sterility of a Turner's type. This entire series of regulatory events occurs only in the female and may represent a unique genetic load that would be expressed in decreased survival of females in utero. In fact, there appear to be more chromosomally normal female abortuses than male (Hassold et al., 1980), and it is possible that part of the well-known excess of males at birth might be due to failure of X inactivation at any one of a number of developmental steps.

ERRORS IN THE MAINTENANCE FEATURES OF X INACTIVATION

In most differentiative steps, selective activation and silencing of particular genes occur in conjunction with a marked reduction or cessation of cell division of the differentiated cells. In X inactivation, which is an intracellular form of differentiation and takes place in all somatic cells, the differential selective silencing and activation of the two X chromosomes must be renewed at every cell division. That is, proper differential methylation must follow each round of DNA replication and the same X chromosome must form sex chromatin after every mitosis. Several possibilities for error exist here and examples of each have now been reported.

Errors here may lead to reactivation on the inactive X chromosome or to inactivation of genes on the active X. The latter could ocur in males as well as females. Because there is only a single active X in the female, inactivation would be expected to have similar effects in male and female cells. However, the presence of the inactive allele in the female raises the possibility, at least, of a compensatory reaction in female cells. Reactivation of X-linked genes can only occur in the female, and the recent report of reactivation of the ornithine transcarbamylase gene in aging mice (Wareham, Lyon, Glenister, & Williams, 1987) has prompted speculation regarding the effect of this event. Some years earlier Cattanach (1974) reported that in aging mice with an X:autosome translocation an inactivated gene on the autosomal segment appeared to undergo reactivation with age. Holliday (1987) has argued that reactivation would impair dosage compensation and be harmful to the female. If reactivation took place at the chromosomal level, then Holliday's interpretation is probably correct, but there is absolutely no evidence for chromosomal reactivation. What the effect of reactivation of individual genes would be is not known, either theoretically or empirically. Besides reactivation, it is also possible to consider inactivation of normally active genes by aberrant spreading of the X-inactivation processes. This event has recently been reported by our laboratory for the murine steroid sulfatase *(STS)* locus that maps in the pairing region of the X and Y chromosomes. It has functional alleles on the X and the Y, is subject to obligatory recombination, and under normal conditions, completely escapes X inactivation. We had observed that established murine cell lines were STS deficient even though some of the lines were known to be derived from STS$^+$ animals. To investigate this phenomenon we developed a selective technique for detecting STS$^+$ revertants occurring in STS$^-$ cultures and were able to demonstrate that STS$^+$ revertants were produced with high frequency after treatment of the STS– cultures with the demethylating agent, 5-azacytidine. The interpretation of this work is that aberrant methylation has spread into a region that normally escapes all aspects of the X-inactivation system. We have been able to recreate the loss of STS activity in cell culture by following new cultures initiated from STS$^+$ embryos and testing their STS activity at frequent transfers. After 80 to 100 cell doublings, STS activity is lost and usually in a rather abrupt manner (Schorderet, Keitges, Dubois, & Gartler, 1988).

Up to this point we have written about methylation as though it was a unique X-chromosome regulatory mechanism. This is clearly not the case. Major attention was drawn to DNA methylation when Riggs (1975) proposed methylation as a candidate for regulatory control, including X-chromosome inactivation. The attraction of methylation as a regulatory system was based on two features: (1) DNA methylation was known to modify DNA binding of regulatory proteins, and (2) methylation kinetics, especially those of the maintenance methylase (methylates half-methylated sites efficiently and unmethylated sites very inefficiently), are ideally suited to maintaining a differentiated state over many cell divisions. This research led to considerable interest in methylation, but the first experimental support for the idea did not appear until 1980 when Jones and Taylor (1980) showed that 5AC treatment of an undifferentiated transformed mouse culture led to the appearance of several differentiated cell types. Within a short time, a number of reports appeared showing the activating effect of 5AC on a number of genes, autosomal as well as X-linked (e.g., thymidine kinase; prolactin; glucocorticord resistance; hepatitis B virus core gene; α-globin; *G6pd; Hprt;* α-galactosidase; and phosphoglycerate kinase) (Harris, 1986; Mohandas, Sparks, & Shapiro, 1981). All of these cases involved cell culture studies, and the 5AC work implied that a number of so-called deficiency mutants were not true mutants, but rather epigenetic in nature, their repression being due to hypermethylation. In those cases where molecular probes became available, it was usually shown that the activated genes had become demethylated in CpG-rich 5' regions. In this same period a number of reports appeared showing a decrease in general DNA methylation level with age (Shmookler Reis, & Goldstein, 1982; Wilson, Smith, Ma, & Cutler, 1987). It was proposed that a component of aging might be attributed to inappropriate activation or reactivation of genes by aberrant demethylation connected with replication and/or DNA repair. Of particular interest was the possibility of activation of oncogenes by demethylation (Mays-Hoopes, Chao, Butcher, & Huang, 1986; Ono, Tawa, Shinya, Hirose, & Okada, 1986). Recent reports of decreases in life span of fibroblast cultures after 5AC treatment have been interpreted as supporting the hypothesis of a correlation, possibly causal, between demethylation and decreased longevity (Fairweather, Fox, & Margison, 1987; Holliday, 1986).

Another aspect of methylation that could be of considerable importance with respect to aging is remethylation. Remethylation can be studied by examining methylation patterns following 5AC induced demethylation. There are two reports of such studies at the molecular level. Faltau and colleagues (1984), using a general methylation assay, reported that transformed mouse cells remethylated their DNA following 5AC treatment, although some variant lines could be obtained that remained at reduced methylation levels. Ley et al. (1984), using gene-specific probes in a mouse–human somatic cell hybrid, reported that following 5AC treatment and demethylation, the human insulin gene was rapidly remethylated while the human globin gene remained demethylated. We have observed in normal human cells, following 5AC treatment, that the 5' ends of the *Pgk* and *Hprt* genes are apparently remethylated following significant demethylation. On the other hand, these same genes in a transformed rodent–human hybrid appear to remain demethylated following 5AC treatment. These latter observations suggest to us that remethylation may depend both on gene and cell type, and this must be considered in any evaluation of the role of demethylation in aging materials.

There is little doubt from the above-mentioned work that methylation of specific regions of many genes can lead to their repression and, likewise, demethylation of the same regions may be a necessary, though not sufficient, condition for expression. What determines normal methylation patterns and causes aberrant ones is not known as yet, though we feel that X-inactivation studies support the notion of chromatin configuration acting as a pattern for proper methylation. Abnormal chromatin configuration could open up the possibility for de novo methylation and aberrant repression or demethylation and aberrant expression. In turn, it could be cell aging that leads to abnormal chromatin structure in some regions.

The methylation studies cited above have also demonstrated a general demethylation that is associated with age. However, there is no definitive evidence as yet that the demethylation associated with aging is involved in aberrant expression or repression of genes. In fact, it is conceivable that most and possibly all of the demethylation that has been observed in aging cells is a necessary part of normal maturation. It must be kept in mind that while most of the C_pGs in mammalian DNA are methylated, there is, at least, indirect evidence that expression control is restricted to methylation in restricted parts of a gene. In other words, it appears that there can be considerable changes in methylation, perhaps in most regions of a gene, without a significant effect on expression.

Aberrant methylation, either de- or hypermethylation, can affect both autosomal and X-linked genes. In the case of an autosomal gene the effect on males and females should be similar. However, for X-linked genes the effects will vary with sex. Demethylation leading to reactivation of genes on the inactive X is restricted to females, and if the entire X chromosome is reactivated, the effect would be damaging to chromosome balance and cell viability. Although, I suspect that this event is very unlikely, reactivation of individual genes on the inactive X does occur and may take place more frequently in aging cells. What effects such reactivation would have on cell function is not immediately apparent, and this question will require experimental work.

Hypermethylation leading to inactivation of X-linked genes would take place on the active X and, therefore, could occur in both males and females. In the case of males such X-chromosomal events would create a deficiency that should, in general, affect cell function. The same should apply to the female, with the exception that the inactive X could conceivably act as a reservoir of potentially reactivatable genes.

In summary, it seems clear that aberrant methylation of X-linked genes occurs with some frequency and is likely to be associated with age. However, it is not at all clear as to whether such events will affect males and females in a significantly different way.

One other type of error that has been reported to occur regarding X inactivation is the association of X-chromosome aneuploidy and age. This was first reported in 1961 (Jacobs, Court Brown, & Doll, 1961) when it was shown that there was a general increase in aneuploidy in aging peripheral blood cells, but that aneuploidy was especially high for X chromosomes. In the majority of cases the X-chromosome aneuploidy involved monosomy and it was assumed that the lost X was the inactive one. This initial observation has been confirmed (Galloway & Buckton, 1978; Nakagome, Abe, Misawa, Takeshita, & Iinuma, 1984), and recently it has been shown by replication studies that in the majority of cases the lost X was indeed the inactive one, but surprisingly some 10% of the monosomic X cells involved loss of the active X chromosome (Abruzzo, Mayer, & Jacob, 1985). Analysis of the trisomy X cells showed that the majority involved duplication of the inactive X, but surprisingly over 20% involved duplication of the active X. Both the monosomic X cells with an inactive X and the trisomic X cells with two active X chromosomes should be extremely unbalanced. The long-term survival of these monosomies (effectively nullisomic) is questionable, and the trisomics with two active Xs could well lead to unbalanced growth.

It would seem that sex chromosome aneuploidy in somatic cells should occur with equal frequency in males and females. Because the males have an active X only, aneuploidies should be more damaging for the male than for the female.

X-LINKED MOSAICISM IN HETEROZYGOTES AND CELL SELECTION

Once X inactivation is established, the female becomes a natural mosaic with some cells expressing the paternal X and others the maternal X. For any heterozygous cell autonomous locus, this mosaicism may be detected by a variety of methods depending on the particular marker. Histochemical methods may be used and single cell differences detected, or single cells may be cloned and grown into sizeable populations for extractive biochemistry. These heterozygous markers are like built-in cell tracers that may be used for developmental studies both abnormal, as in tumor tracking (Linder & Gartler, 1965), and for normal embryology, as in determining embryonic stem pool sizes

(Nesbitt & Gartler, 1971). The mosaic nature of the female for X-linked genes also means that cell selection is possible. Somatic selection in X-linked heterozygotes was first demonstrated in cell culture some years ago using the glucose-6-phosphate dehydrogenase (G6PD) Mediterranean variants (Gartler & Linder, 1964). Heterozygous cultures showing initially an approximately 50:50 composition became 100% deficient after a number of doublings. Later this study was repeated with G6PD electrophoretic variants (A and B) and again selection was demonstrated with cultures usually beginning at 50A:50B, and ending up either 100%A or 100%B (Zavala, Herner, & Fialkow, 1978). The pattern of approach to fixation was repeatable in duplications of the same culture. These are clear demonstrations of cell selection occurring in these mosaic cultures, though it is unlikely that selection is acting on the G6PD locus. It is more likely that this locus is merely serving as a marker to detect selection. Selection appears to act on almost every culture in which mosaicism can be detected.

Is it possible that selection also takes place in vivo? Definitive evidence for selection in vivo comes from observations on individuals heterozygous for the Lesch-Nyhan disease [hypoxanthine phosphoribosyltransferase (HPRT) deficiency]. Such females, who are phenotypically normal, show a nonmosaic pattern in their hematopoietic cells with all cells being HPRT$^+$, while skin samples show the typical mosaic pattern found in most individuals heterozygous for X-linked genes (a mixture of HPRT$^+$ and HPRT$^-$ cells) (Nyhan, Bakay, Connor, Marks, & Keele, 1970). Selection in this case is acting on the HPRT system and selecting for HPRT activity at the cellular level in blood but not solid tissues. This same phenomenon has also been reported for several X-linked immune deficiency syndromes (Conley et al., 1986; Prchal et al., 1980). Another more general adaptive response due to selection in X-inactivation mosaic systems relates to observations on individuals heterozygous for X-chromosome abnormalities (deletions, duplications, translocations). In such cases the final pattern of X inactivation is one that represents the most balanced chromosomal composition possible. For example, in reciprocal X:autosome translocations the intact X is nearly always the inactivated chromosome (Keitges & Palmer, 1986). Initially, inactivation is random, but those cells in which the rearranged X is inactivated are selected against due to resulting chromosome imbalance (double expression of the noninactivated X segment and effective autosomal monosomy due to spreading of inactivation). Possibly the best illustration of the adaptive nature of such selection is a case of an interstitial duplication of the X representing less than 10% of the chromosome. The male with such a duplication shows a marked aneuploidy effect but the heterozygous female appears completely normal due to elimination of those cells in which the normal X was inactivated. Studies of population samples of known heterozygotes for G6PD variation have consistently shown a few percent to be nonmosaic in their red blood cells. These studies have been carried out in populations in which malaria and/or favism have been present, and it is possible that some of the apparent selection in red blood cells could represent adaptive changes in cell composition. Somatic cell selection based on X-chromosome mosaicism can only occur in females and it seems that in most, if not all, cases studied so far the selection is adaptive. Such adaptive somatic cell selection occurring in inactivation mosaics could contribute to the known gender age gap.

Studies of cell selection for X-linked mosaics are restricted to heterozygotes and have been limited in the past because of the small number of X-linked polymorphisms. The availability of restriction fragment length polymorphisms in conjunction with 5' methylation differences at X-linked housekeeping genes means that X-linked heterozygotes are now widely available and should no longer limit such studies (Fearon, Hamilton, & Vogelstein, 1987).

CONCLUSION

Years ago Ashley Montague pointed to the 2X:1X chromosome difference between the sexes as a possible explanation of the gender difference in longevity. At that time we were unaware of the phenomenon of X-chromosome inactivation and it has been the purpose here to consider the implications of X inactivation for the question of the gender difference in longevity.

Three ways in which X inactivation might affect the sexes in a differential manner have been pointed out. First, the embryology of X inactivation may be considered as a developmental load unique to the female, and, consequently, any aberrations in the system would affect females more than males. Though the consequences of such aberrations might ultimately contribute to the sex ratio difference at birth, the gender longevity difference would not be affected.

Secondly, once X-chromosome inactivation is established it must be maintained at every cell division. As with any complicated biological system, given enough time, it is certain that errors will occur and we are already aware of reactivation and inactivation of previously inactive and active genes. Part of the maintenance system is DNA methylation, and it is clear that methylation errors in both directions can take place and at least, in some instances, bring about changes in expression. While it is certain that errors in maintenance of X inactivation are occurring, their extent and significance for the question of the gender difference in longevity are not at all clear.

Finally, the mosaic nature of the female, which is a natural result of the X-inactivation process, may have considerable relevance to the gender longevity difference. Mosaicism means that cell selection is possible, and many instances of such selection have been reported. In a number of these cases selection appears to be adaptive, and because X-chromosome-related mosaicism and selection can only occur in the female, it is possible that this aspect of X inactivation may contribute to the gender longevity difference.

REFERENCES

Abruzzo, M. A., Mayer, M., & Jacob, P. A. (1985). Aging and aneuploidy: Evidence for the preferential involvement of the inactive X chromosome. *Cytogenetics and Cell Genetics, 39,* 275–278.

Cattanach, B. M. (1974). Position effect variegation in the mouse. *Genetical Research, 23,* 291–306.

Conley, M. E., Brown, P., Pickard, A. R., Buckley, R. H., Miller, D. S., Raskind, W. H., Singer, J. W., & Fialkow, P. J. (1986). Expression of the gene defect in X-linked agammaglobulinemia. *The New England Journal of Medicine, 315,* 564–567.

Fairweather, D. S., Fox, M., & Margison, G. P. (1987). The in vitro lifespan of MRC-5 cells is shortened by 5-azacytidine-induced demethylation. *Experimental Cell Research, 168,* 153–159.

Fearon, E. R., Hamilton, S. R., & Vogelstein, B. (1987). Clonal analysis of human colorectal tumors. *Science, 238,* 193–197.

Flatau, E., Gonzales, F. A., Michalowsky, L. A., & Jones, P. A. (1984). DNA methylation in 5-aza-2'-deoxycytidine-resistant variants of C3H 10T½ C18 cells. *Molecular and Cellular Biology, 4,* 2098–2102.

Galloway, S. M., & Buckton, K. E. (1978). Aneuploidy and ageing: Chromosome studies on a random sample of the population using G-banding. *Cytogenetics and Cell Genetics, 20,* 78–95.

Gartler, S. M., Dyer, K. A., Graves, J. A. M., & Rocchi, M. (1985). A two step model for mammalian X-chromosome inactivation. In G. L. Cantoni & A. Razin (Eds.), *Biochemistry and biology of DNA methylation* (pp. 223–232). New York: Liss.

Gartler, S. M., & Linder, D. (1964). Selection in mammalian mosaic cell Populations. *Cold Spring Harbor Symposia on Quantitative Biology, 29,* 253–260.

Gartler, S. M., & Riggs, A. D. (1983). Mammalian X-chromosome inactivation. *Annual Review of Genetics, 17,* 155–190.

Harris, M. (1986). Induction and reversion of asparagine auxotrophs in CHO-K1 and V79 cells. *Somatic Cell and Molecular Genetics, 12,* 459–466.

Hassold, T., Chen, N., Funkhouser, J., Jooss, T., Manuel, B., Matsuura, J., Matsuyama, A., Wilson, C., Yamane, J. A., & Jacobs, P. A. (1980). A cytogenetic study of 1000 spontaneous abortions. *Annals of Human Genetics, 44,* 151–178.

Holliday, R. (1986). Strong effects of 5-azacytidine on the in vitro lifespan of human diploid fibroblasts. *Experimental Cell Research, 166,* 543–552.

Holliday, R. (1987). X-chromosome reactivation. *Nature, 327,* 661–662.

Jacobs, P. A., Court Brown, W. M., & Doll, R. (1961). Distribution of human chromosome counts in relation to age. *Nature, 191,* 1178–1180.

Jones, P. A., & Taylor, S. M. (1980). Cellular differentiation, cytidine analogs and DNA methylation. *Cell, 20,* 85–93.

Keitges, E. A., & Palmer, C. G. (1986). Analysis of spreading of inactivation in eight X autosome translocations utilizing the high resolution RBG technique. *Human Genetics, 72,* 231–236.

Keitges, E. A., Schorderet, D. F., & Gartler, S. M. (1987). Linkage of the steroid sulfatase gene to the *sex-reversed* mutation in the mouse. *Genetics, 116,* 465–468.

Kratzer, P. G., Chapman, V. M., Lambert, H., Evans, R. E., & Liskay, R. M. (1983). Differences in the DNA of the inactive X chromosomes of fetal and extraembryonic tissues of mice. *Cell, 33,* 37–42.

Ley, T. J., Chiang, Y. L., Haidaris, D., Anagnou, N. P., Wilson, V. L., & Anderson, W. F. (1984). DNA methylation and regulation of the human β-globin-like genes in mouse erythroleukemia cells containing human chromosome 11. *Proceedings of the National Academy of Sciences USA, 81,* 6618–6622.

Linder, D., & Gartler, S. M. (1965). Glucose-6-phosphate dehydrogenase mosaicism: Utilization as a cell marker in the study of leiomyomas. *Science, 150,* 67–69.

Lock, L. F. Takagi, N., & Martin, G. R. (1987). Methylation of the *Hprt* gene on the inactive X occurs after chromosome inactivation. *Cell, 48,* 39–46.

Lyon, M. F. (1961). Gene action in the X-chromosome of the mouse (*Mus musculus* L.). *Nature, 190,* 372–373.

Mays-Hoopes, L., Chao, W., Butcher, H. C., & Huang, R. C. C. (1986). Decreased methylation of the major mouse long interspersed repeated DNA during aging and in myeloma cells. *Developmental Genetics, 7,* 65–73.

Mohandas, T., Sparkes, R. S., & Shapiro, L. J. (1981). Reactivation of an inactive human X chromosome: Evidence for X inactivation by DNA methylation. *Science, 211,* 393–396.

Muller, H. J., League, B. B., & Offerman, C. A. (1931). Effects of dosage changes of sex-linked genes, and the compensatory effects of other gene differences between male and female (Abstract). *The Anatomical Record, 51,* 110.

Nakagome, Y., Abe, T., Misawa, S., Takeshita, T., & Iinuma, K. (1984). The "loss" of centromeres from chromosomes of aged women. *The American Journal of Human Genetics, 36,* 398–404.

Nesbitt, M. N., & Gartler, S. M. (1971). The applications of genetic mosaicism to developmental problems. *Annual Review of Genetics, 5,* 143–162.

Nyhan, W. L., Bakay, B., Connor, J. D., Marks, J. F., & Keele, D. K. (1970). Hemizygous expression of glucose-6-phosphate dehydrogenase in erythrocytes of heterozygotes for the Lesch-Nyan syndrome. *Proceedings of the National Academy of Sciences USA, 65,* 214–218.

Ono, T., Tawa, R., Shinya, K., Hirose, S., & Okada, S. (1986). Methylation of the c-myc gene changes during aging process of mice. *Biochemical and Biophysical Research Communications, 139,* 1299–1304.

Prchal, J. T., Carroll, A. J., Prchal, J. F., Crist, W. M., Skalka, H. W., Gealy, W. J., Harley, J., & Malluh, A. (1980). Wiskott-Aldrich syndrome: Cellular impairments and their implication for carrier detection. *Blood, 56,* 1048–1054.

Riggs, A. D. (1975). X inactivation, differentiation, and DNA methylation. *Cytogenetics and Cell Genetics, 14,* 9–25.

Riggs, A. D. Singer-Sam, J., & Keith, D. H. (1985). Methylation of the PGK promoter region and an enhancer way-station model for X-chromosome inactivation. In G. L. Cantoni & A. Razin (Eds.), *Biochemistry and biology of DNA methylation* (pp. 211–222). New York: Liss.

Riley, D. E., Goldman, M. A., & Gartler, S. M. (1986). Chromatin structure of active and inactive human X-linked phosphoglycerate kinase gene. *Somatic Cell and Molecular Genetics, 12,* 73–80.

Rouyer, F., Simmler, M. C., Johnsson, C., Vergnaud, G., Cooke, H. J., & Weissenbach, J. (1986). A gradient of sex linkage in the pseudoautosomal region of the human sex chromosomes. *Nature, 319,* 291–295.

Schorderet, D. F., Keitges, E. A., Dubois, P. M., & Gartler, S. M. (1988). Inactivation and reactivation of sex-linked steroid sulfatase gene in murine cell culture. *Somatic Cell and Molecular Genetics, 14,* 113–121.

Shmookler Reis, R. J., & Goldstein, S. (1982). Variability of DNA methylation patterns during serial passage of human diploid fibroblasts. *Proceedings of the National Academy of Sciences USA, 79,* 3949–3953.

Toniolo, D., Martini, G., Migeon, B. R., & Dono, R. (1988). Expression of the G6PD locus on the human X chromosome is associated with demethylation of three CpG islands within 100 kb of DNA. *The EMBO Journal, 7,* 401–406.

Wareham, K. A., Lyon, M. F., Glenister, P. H., & Williams, E. D. (1987). Age related reactivation of an X-linked gene. *Nature, 327,* 725–727.

Wilson, V. L., Smith, R. A., Ma, S., & Cutler, R. G. (1987). Genomic 5-methyldeoxycytidine decreases with age. *The Journal of Biological Chemistry, 262,* 9948–9951.

Wolf, S. F., Jolly, D. J., Lunnen, K. D., Friedmann, T., & Migeon, B. R. (1984). Methylation of the hypoxanthine phosphoribosyltransferase locus on the human X chromosome: implications for X-chromosome inactivation. *Proceedings of the National Academy of Sciences USA, 81,* 2806–2810.

Zavala, C., Herner, G., & Fialkow, P. J. (1978). Evidence for selection in cultured diploid fibroblast strains. *Experimental Cell Research, 117,* 137–144.

6 A Central Role of Sex Hormones in the Sex Differential in Lipoprotein Metabolism, Atherosclerosis, and Longevity

William R. Hazzard

Insight into the sex differential in human longevity (Hazzard, 1986) begins with inspection of the leading causes of death in Occidental society, the contribution that elimination of each of these might make to increasing longevity (Table 6.1), and the sex differential in each of these causes (Table 6.2). While such a pervasive biological phenomenon as greater female longevity is certain to prove of complex causality, such analysis places atherosclerosis and its complications, notably coronary heart disease, stroke, and other sequelae, squarely in focus. Thus, the combination of the high probability of death from cardiovascular disease with the nearly 2:1 male:female ratio in such mortality clearly suggests that the sex differential in atherosclerosis may constitute the largest single cause of the sex differential in longevity in contemporary American society.

GENDER DIFFERENTIALS IN CIGARETTE SMOKING AND ITS DISEASE CONSEQUENCES

Like all chronic diseases of middle and old age, atherosclerotic cardiovascular disease is multifactorial in origin. An overarching consideration in the sex differential in longevity related not only to atherosclerosis, but also to other leading causes of death in middle and old age has been the historical sex differential in cigarette smoking. Among the 12 leading causes of death (Table 6.2), this cigarette smoking behavioral differential could clearly contribute to higher male

Table 6.1 Gain in Expectation of Life at Birth and at the Age of 65 Due to Elimination of Various Causes of Death.*

Cause of Death	Gain (Yr) in Expectation of Life if Cause was Eliminated	
	At Birth	At Age of 65
Major cardiovascular-renal diseases	10.9	10.0
Heart diseases	5.9	4.9
Vascular diseases affecting central nervous system	1.3	1.2
Malignant neoplasms	2.3	1.2
Accidents, excluding those caused by motor vehicles	0.6	0.1
Motor-vehicle accidents	0.6	0.1
Influenza & pneumonia	0.5	0.2
Infectious diseases (excluding tuberculosis)	0.2	0.1
Diabetes mellitus	0.2	0.2
Tuberculosis	0.1	0.0

*Source: Life tables published by National Center of Health Statistics, US Public Health Service & US Bureau of Census, "Some Demographic Aspects of Aging in the United States," February, 1973.

mortality in several categories: heart disease, malignant neoplasms, cerebrovascular diseases, chronic obstructive lung disease, pneumonia and influenza, diabetes mellitus (given that atherosclerotic complications are the leading causes of death in diabetics), and atherosclerosis of noncardiac varieties. Indeed, a consensus among experts suggests that this traditional sex differential in cigarette smoking may account for as much as four of the seven years in the overall sex differential in longevity that characterizes the present era (Holden, 1983). Since the Surgeon General's Report on Smoking and Health of 1963, cigarette smoking has declined in both males and females in the United States (just as cardiovascular mortality has declined in both males and females). While in both instances the relative (percentage) decreases in cigarette smoking have been similar in men and women, the absolute declines have been greater in men than in women. Hence, it is not surprising that recent trends in such clear-cut consequences of cigarette abuse as lung cancer suggest a narrowing in the sex differential in this disease and, in turn, the prospect that other diseases related to cigarette smoking may also narrow in their sex differential as cigarette smoking behavior in women comes more closely to resemble that of men.

Table 6.2 Sex-specific mortality rates and sex differentials for the twelve leading causes of death,[a] United States, 1980[b]

Cause	Age-adjusted mortality rate[c]		Sex ratio (M/F)	Sex difference (M–F)
	Males	Females		
Diseases of the heart	280.4	140.3	1.99	140.1
Malignant neoplasms	165.5	109.2	1.51	56.3
Respiratory system	59.7	18.3	3.43	41.4
Cerebrovascular diseases	44.9	37.6	1.19	7.3
Accidents	64.0	21.8	2.93	42.2
Motor vehicle	34.3	11.8	2.90	22.5
Other	29.6	10.0	2.96	19.6
Chronic obstructive pulmonary disease	26.1	8.9	2.93	17.2
Pneumonia and influenza	17.4	9.8	1.77	7.6
Diabetes mellitus	10.2	10.0	1.02	0.2
Cirrhosis of the liver	17.1	7.9	2.16	9.2
Atherosclerosis	6.6	5.0	1.32	1.6
Suicide	18.0	5.4	3.33	12.6
Homicide	17.4	4.5	3.86	12.9
Certain causes in infancy	11.1	8.7	1.27	2.4
All causes	777.2	432.6	1.79	344.6

[a]Rank based on number of deaths.
[b]Calculated from data from the National Center for Health Statistics, 1983.
[c]Per 100,000, direct standardization to the 1940 total US population.

Source: Reprinted with permission from D. L. Wingard, The sex differential in morbidity, mortality and lifestyle. *Ann Rev Pub Health, 5,* pp. 433–458, 1984.

ROLE OF SEX HORMONES IN SEX DIFFERENTIAL IN ATHEROSCLEROSIS

Another primary hypothesis requiring careful assessment is that sex hormones may play a fundamental role in the sex differential in chronic diseases, notably atherosclerosis. Evaluation of this possibility begins with analysis of the sex differential in adult cardiovascular mortality with advancing age (Figure 6.1). This discloses a dramatic differential in young and middle age, the sex ratio (M:F) declining with increasing age throughout the remainder of adult life (though the ratio never reaches unity, even in advanced old age). These same data can be viewed more traditionally, by gender, as a function of increasing age beyond 35 years (Figure 6.2). This depiction reveals an exponential rise in ischemic heart disease deaths with advancing age in both genders; however, the rate in females lags approximately a de-

Genetic and Biologic Bases

Figure 6.1 Linear sex ratio (M:F) in cardiovascular mortality, coronary and hypertensive, in the United States, by age and race, 1955.

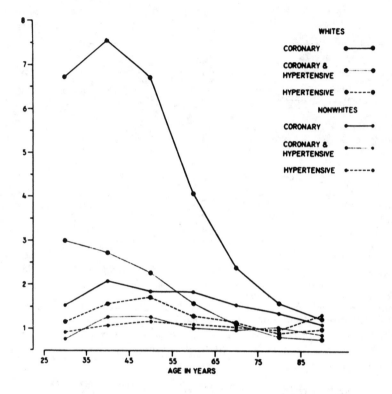

From Furman, R. H. (1973). Coronary heart disease and the menopause. In K. J. Ryan, & D. C. Gibson, (Eds.), Menopause and Aging. US Department of HEW, DHEW Publication No. [NIH] 73–319.

cade behind that in males across the entire adult life span. Hence, the average woman enjoys an approximately ten year relative immunity to death from ischemic heart disease compared with her male counterparts, presumably by virtue of her gender and, perhaps, the sex differential in the sex hormones. Interestingly, a similar Gestalt is seen with regard to the percentage cumulative heart disease incidence even among those uncommon persons (ca. 1 in 500) who have inherited a major cause for vastly premature atherosclerosis, specifically, familial hypercholesterolemia, based in a heterozygously determined deficiency of the receptor for the low-density lipoprotein (LDL) (Figure

Figure 6.2 Death rates per 100,000 population for ischemic heart disease by age in years in men (closed circles) and women (open circles) in the United States in 1976.

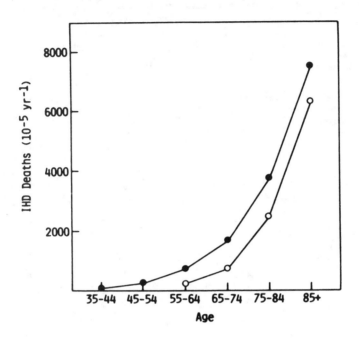

Reprinted with permission from J. L. Sullivan. (1983). The sex differential in ischemic heart disease. *Perspectives in Biology and Medicine, 26,* p. 658.

6.3). Thus, women who share this genetic disorder with their brothers still enjoy an approximately ten year immunity from the complications of their high levels of LDL cholesterol.

The next level of insight comes from inspection of ischemic heart disease incidence among women who are pre- versus those of comparable age who are post-menopausal. Data displayed in Figure 6.4 in semilogarithmic fashion, which linearizes the increased ischemic heart disease mortality incidence with age in both genders, suggest that post-menopausal women have a substantially higher risk of cardiovascular disease than do women of the same age with intact ovarian function (they are still at lower risk, however, than men of comparable age). These data clearly imply a significant role for sex steroid hormones in the relative immunity of women to premature ischemic heart disease compared to their male counterparts.

Figure 6.3 Percentage of cumulative incidence of first attack from ischemic heart disease by age in years in men (closed circles) and women (open circles) heterozygous for familial hypercholesterolemia (Fredrickson's type II hyperbetalipoproteinemia).

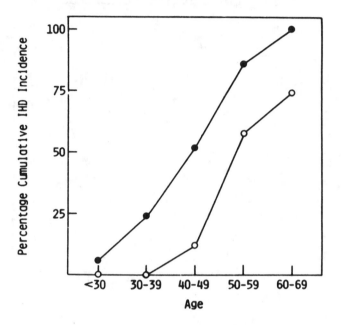

Reprinted with permission from J. L. Sullivan. (1983). The sex differential in ischemic heart disease. *Perspectives in Biology and Medicine, 26,* p. 665.

GENDER DIFFERENTIALS IN MAJOR CHD RISK FACTORS

The next level of inquiry requires consideration by gender of a hierarchy of cardiovascular risk attributes in middle and old age in both univariate and, more importantly, multivariate fashion. Those from a recent analysis of the longitudinal Framingham Study (Table 6.3) place high-density lipoprotein (HDL) cholesterol as by far the most powerful factor, except that this is in an inverse fashion; that is, high HDL cholesterols are associated with low cardiovascular disease risk, while low HDL cholesterols are associated with high cardiovascular risk. Interestingly, the apparent sex differential in the power of this inverse relationship seen on univariate analysis disappears on multivariate analysis. Second in power of prediction is the LDL cholesterol,

Figure 6.4 Incidence of cardiovascular disease by age in years, sex, and menopausal status in the Framingham Study 20-year follow-up. Rates per 1000 per year are displayed for men (closed circles), all women (open circles), premenopausal women (downward arrowhead), and postmenopausal women (upward arrowhead). Rates for pre- and post-menopausal women "less than 40 years" are plotted with the 35 to 39 year group.

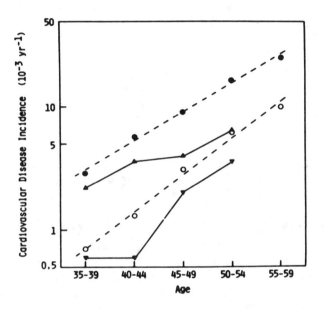

Reprinted with permission from J. L. Sullivan. (1983). The sex differential in ischemic heart disease. *Perspectives in Biology and Medicine, 26,* p. 661.

in the expected positive fashion. Triglyceride levels, which on univariate analysis appear to be a risk index in women only, become nonsignificant on multivariate analysis. Systolic blood pressure is a positive risk attribute in both genders, though weaker in women on multivariate analysis. Left ventricular hypertrophy is a relatively weak positive index in both genders. Relative weight, like triglyceride, appears on univariate analysis to be a risk index in women only, but this disappears on multivariate analysis. In both instances, this is attributed to the inverse relationship between both triglyceride level and relative weight and the HDL cholesterol; that is, the reduction in HDL cholesterol associated with increases in both triglyceride and relative weight appears to be the proximate mediator of increased risk associated with these characteristics. Viewed in a different way, in the

Table 6.3 Coefficient for Regression of CHD Incidence of Risk Factors Men and Women 50 to 82 Years Framingham Study

| | Standardized logistic regression coefficients | | | |
| | Univariate | | Multivariate | |
Risk attributes	Men	Women	Men	Women
HDL cholesterol	−.488*	−.741	−.610*	−.650
LDL cholesterol	.288[†]	.303[†]	.332[‡]	.260[†]
Triglyceride	.048	.276	−.092	−.106
Systolic pressure	.323[‡]	.400[‡]	.327[‡]	.216
ECG-LVH	.279*	.207[‡]	.245[‡]	.159[†]
Relative weight	.029	.283[†]	−.016	.031
Diabetes	−.024	.474*	−.114	.390*

*$p = < .001$.
[†]$p = < .05$.
[‡]$p = < .01$.

Reprinted with permission from W. B. Kannel & F. N. Brand. (1984). Cardiovascular risk factors in the elderly. In R. Andres, E. Bierman, & W. Hazzard (Eds.), *Principles of Geriatric Medicine*, p. 108. New York: McGraw Hill.

overweight, hypertriglyceridemic woman whose HDL remains normal, there would be no associated increased risk of heart disease attributed to either her obesity or hypertriglyceridemia per se. Diabetes mellitus, curiously enough, remains a powerful risk index in women on both univariate and multivariate analysis, while it was not associated with increased risk in middle and old age in men from the Framingham Study. This is a specific exception to the general increase in risk of mortality from all causes in men relative to women (evident in Table 6.2); stated somewhat differently, diabetes is a far more ominous disease in a woman than in a man, because it overrides the relative immunity to cardiovascular and other diseases that she would normally enjoy by virtue of her gender.

SEX DIFFERENTIAL IN LYPOPROTEIN LIPID LEVELS DURING ADULTHOOD

To carry this analysis one step further, let us ask whether average levels of these two leading risk indices, the LDL and HDL cholesterol (and a simple and legitimate shorthand for both in the ratio between the two), themselves change with age during adult life and whether or not such changes in turn might explain the differential in lipoprotein metabolism and associated atherosclerosis. Fortunately, the collaborative Lipid Research Clinics hyperlipidemia prevalence surveys of the 1970s are available to assess LDL, HDL and LDL/HDL data from childhood through early old age in a contemporary 11-community population study (Figure 6.5). Inspection of these data, in which each point represents average values among a large number of participants, shows no differential in LDL, HDL or the ratio between the two until puberty. During adolescence, however, changes between the sexes begin to be expressed. LDL levels rise progressively between puberty and the era of the menopause in both genders, but rise faster and remain higher in men than women throughout this age span; however, across the menopausal era average LDL cholesterol levels increase significantly in women such that mean concentrations in postmeno-pausal women exceed those in men of comparable age. Regarding HDL, a different pattern is evident. Across puberty there occurs a sharp decline in average HDL concentration in boys, while HDL re-mains stable in girls. Moreover, HDL levels remain lower in males than in females throughout the rest of adult life (though there is an intriguing rise among men beyond the menopausal era, conceivably related to declining testicular androgen production). Yet to be con-firmed in specific analyses is the suggestion from these trends that the major hormone responsible for lower LDL levels in women than men from puberty to the menopause is estrogen, its decline across the menopause being responsible for the higher levels of LDL cholesterol in postmenopausal women. In contrast, the lower HDL levels in males beyond puberty would likely be attributable to the effects of an-drogens, given their continued secretion throughout adult life. The net effect of these two trends, given the greater impact in the males of lower HDL levels than in women (who have higher LDL levels in the postmenopausal era) is a continued higher LDL/HDL cholesterol ratio in males and females from puberty throughout adult life. However, an intriguing narrowing in this ratio beyond the menopause is evident.

One might then ask, is the sex differential in these lipoprotein lipid levels sufficient to account for the entire sex differential in atherosclerotic cardiovascular disease? Data to answer this question are limited but suggest that this represents only a partial explanation (Figure 6.6). In this analysis, also from the Framingham Study, in the first three quintiles of total/HDL cholesterol ratio (as a surrogate for the LDL/HDL ratio), at a given ratio males continue to have approx-imately twice the cardiovascular disease incidence of females. On the other hand, in the upper two quintiles of this ratio, quintiles in which well over half of the cardiovascular disease incidence occurs, women are at at the same cardiovascular disease risk as males. Thus, the sex differential in total/HDL cholesterol ratio (or, presumably, LDL/HDL

Figure 6.5 Gender differences in serum cholesterol levels. The figure includes the levels of low density lipoprotein (LDL) cholesterol (top) in men (triangles) and in women (circles); the levels of high density lipoprotein (HDL) cholesterol (middle); and the LDL/HDL ratio (bottom). Plotted are the average values found in the North American population by the Lipid Research Clinic Prevalence Survey.

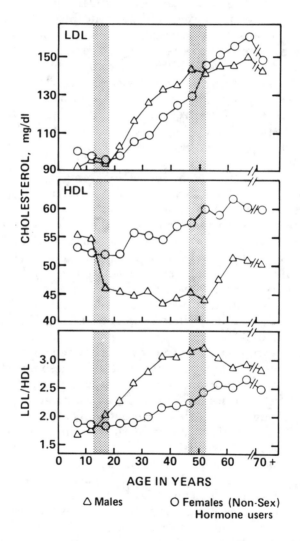

Figure 6.6 Risk of coronary heart disease by total/HDL cholesterol. Framingham study: 26-year follow-up; subjects 50 to 90 years of age.

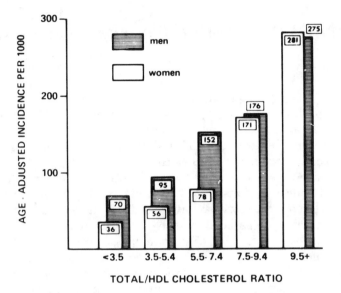

Reprinted with permission from W. B. Kannel & F. N. Brand (1984). Cardiovascular risk factors in the elderly. In R. Andres, E. Bierman, & W. Hazzard (Eds.), *Principles of geratric medicine,* p. 109. New York: McGraw Hill.

ratio) may account for the majority of the sex differential in cardiovascular disease beyond the age 50.

To summarize to this point, the following observations appear to hold true:

1. The male/female coronary risk ratio is greater than 1.0 at all ages (though it narrows progressively with age).
2. The male/female LDL/HDL-cholesterol ratio is also greater than unity at all ages (though it, too, narrows progressively with age):
   a. The male LDL is greater than the female LDL from puberty to menopause (though this pattern is reversed after menopause).
   b. The female HDL is greater than the male HDL from puberty throughout adult life.

Therefore, if one can accept the (perhaps contentious) assumption that men and women share a common life-style, the central hypothesis of this treatise becomes straightforward; that is, the sex differential in sex hormones → sex differential in lipoprotein metabolism → sex differential in atherosclerosis → sex differential in longevity.

LIPOPROTEIN EFFECTS OF EXOGENOUS SEX STEROIDS

Are there any data in support of this simplistic hypothesis? While imperfect and limited, those that are available are generally supportive. Perhaps the most persuasive also come from the Lipid Research Clinics hyperlipidemia prevalence studies, in which a substantial proportion of female participants were taking exogenous sex hormone supplements in the form of combination oral contraceptives or, postmenopausally, estrogens alone. As can be appreciated from Figure 6.7, oral contraceptives appeared to have quite a different effect on cholesterol concentrations than estrogens alone. Oral contraceptives were associated with increased average LDL cholesterol levels, while estrogens alone were associated with clearly decreased concentrations compared in both instances with women taking neither form of hormone supplement. It is readily deduced that this difference is explained by the progestational component of the combination oral contraceptives, such progestins most often being of androgenic origin (19-nortesterone derivatives), with residual androgenic effects. These androgenic effects of the combination oral contraceptives are also evident in the data relating mean HDL cholesterol concentrations to hormone use status in the same female cohort (Figure 6.7). Whereas the use of estrogen alone in postmenopausal women was associated with a clear increase in mean HDL cholesterol concentration, that among combination oral contraceptive users was equivalent to that in nonhormone users. However, when examined yet more carefully, given the wide variety of oral contraceptives used by study participants, those consuming oral contraceptives with a high androgenic progestin/ estrogen relationship had suppressed HDL cholesterol levels, while those taking birth control pills with a weak androgenic progestin/ strong estrogen ratio had HDL cholesterol levels increased above the average in nonhormone taking women (Knopp et al., 1981).

ESTROGEN SUPPLEMENTATION IN
METABOLICALLY-CONTROLLED STUDIES

Additional, direct data in support of a major effect of sex steroids on lipoprotein lipid levels in humans are limited, yet also consistent (Bradley, Wingard, Petit, Krauss, & Ramcharan, 1978; Knopp et al.,

Figure 6.7 Plasma lipoprotein cholesterol levels in users and nonusers of oral contraceptives and estrogens.

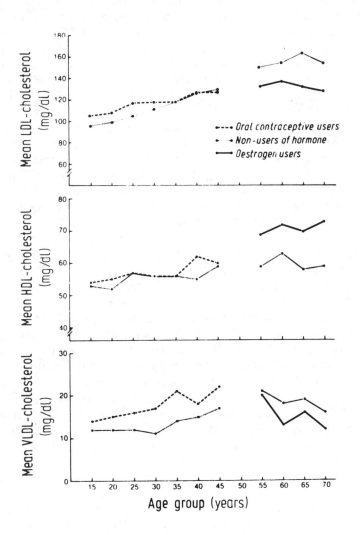

Reprinted with permission from R. B. Wallace et al. (1979). Altered plasma lipid and lipoprotein levels associated with oral contraceptive and oestrogen use. *Lancet, II,* p.1113.

1981; Wahl et al., 1983). When, however, we inspected the literature to determine whether investigators had specifically tested the effect of exogenous sex steroids on lipoprotein metabolism under carefully controlled conditions of constant diet and exercise status, we were surprised to find a dearth of such standardized studies. Therefore, to test the hypothesis that women can tolerate a diet high in cholesterol better than their male counterparts as long as their estrogenic status was maintained, we recruited 6 clearly estrogen-deficient, postmenopausal women (aged 57 ± 6 years) for an 84-day clinical trial of the effect of exogenous estrogen while they consumed an isocaloric (weight-maintaining) diet enriched in cholesterol yet of constant composition (Applebaum-Bowden et al., 1989). This diet, provided in the form of already-prepared meals on an every third day rotating menu, contained 900 mg of added egg yolk cholesterol for a total of approximately 1,000 mg cholesterol per day, roughly 4 times the subjects' normal daily cholesterol intake. To avoid the confounding effects of possible changes in the distribution and quality of calories ingested, the subjects were maintained on a diet of 15% protein, 45% carbohydrate, and 40% fat throughout (with a constant, relatively high polyunsaturated/saturated fat ratio of 0.85). In the middle 28 days of this 84 day trial, the subjects received the oral semisynthetic estrogen, ethinyl estradiol, in a moderately high dose of 1mcg/kg/day. Lipids [triglycerides, cholesterol, total and in LDL, HDL, and the HDL subfractions HDL_2 and HDL_3, the major apolipoprotein carriers in very low density lipoproteins (VLDL) and LDL (B and E) and HDL (A-1 and A-2)], and an enzyme released in the plasma by low doses of heparin, hepatic triglyceride lipase (HTGL), were measured at weekly intervals for the first 28 days prior to the institution of estrogen therapy, at daily intervals during the early phase of estrogen, at increasing intervals in the middle phase, and once again at daily intervals after the estrogen was discontinued, and thereafter at increasing intervals for an additional 28 days.

What were the principal findings of this study? First, surprisingly, lipid levels remained constant during the initial 28 days of the cholesterol-enriched diet: there were no changes in average concentrations of triglyceride or total, LDL or HDL cholesterol. Second, when the estrogen was begun, as predicted, triglyceride levels increased briskly, by approximately 40%, and remained elevated until the estrogen was withdrawn, after which they declined rapidly to baseline levels. Regarding cholesterol levels, surprisingly the total and, specifically, the LDL cholesterol concentration declined briskly during the first several days of estrogen therapy, reaching a nadir by the end of the 4th day and remaining at that depressed level throughout the 28 days of estrogen, rebounding rapidly thereafter to pre-estrogen levels. HDL, on the other hand, increased gradually and progressively after an initial delay of several days, reaching an apparent plateau shortly before the estrogen was withdrawn, declining relatively slowly toward baseline after estrogen was discontinued. The major apolipoprotein carriers followed their parent lipoprotein classes in consistent fashion; apo B declined 11% (presumably reflecting a selective decrease in LDL apo B), while apo E decreased by 36%, both remaining depressed throughout estrogen therapy and then rebounding to preestrogen levels. The major HDL apolipoproteins A-1 and A-2 showed contrasting responses: A-1 increased in parallel with HDL cholesterol levels, while A-2 remained constant during estrogen therapy. Perhaps most telling, the LDL/HDL ratio declined by an average of 40%, from a level of approximately 2.5 prior to estrogen therapy (a value of 3.0 is commonly perceived as the threshold for concern regarding atherogenic risk) to a remarkably low figure of approximately 1.5 during estrogen therapy, increasing gradually to baseline after estrogen was discontinued.

The absolute levels of cholesterol were of significant interest, particularly in light of the current emphasis on maintaining acceptable cholesterol concentrations in the interest of minimizing cardiovascular disease risk (Table 6.4). The mean total cholesterol concentration in these postmenopausal women, approximately 255 mg/100 ml, was in the range wherein at least dietary therapy would currently be recommended. However, in spite of a diet yet further enriched in cholesterol, during estrogen therapy the women's average LDL levels, which were increased above the population 90th percentile prior to therapy, declined to the middle of the clearly acceptable range at 130 mg/100 ml during therapy. Moreover, their HDL-cholesterol levels, high before theapy at approximately 70 mg/100 ml (a concentration of 55 would be expected in average adult women), increased yet further, this increase being confined to the putatively, most antiatherogenic subfraction, HDL_2 (Eder, 1979). Thus, in these normolipidemic postmenopausal women supplemented with oral semisynthetic estrogen, in spite of a diet high in cholesterol, the LDL/HDL ratio remained in a range placing them within the lowest quintile of cardiovascular risk according to current recommended guidelines. Put another way, the estrogen had a more profound effect in altering the LDL/HDL ratio than any hypolipidemic agent currently available, including the recently released HMG CoA reductase inhibitors.

Finally, estrogen therapy was associated with a uniform, brisk, and profound reduction in the activity of HTGL, mean levels being depressed by approximately 70% throughout, returning rapidly to base-

Table 6.4 Mean Cholesterol Level Changes During a Fixed High Cholesterol Diet and with the Addition of Estrogent in Postmenopausal Women*

Day	Cholesterol (mg/dL)					
	Total	VLDL	IDL + LDL	HDL	HDL_2	HDL_3
0	256 ± 36	14 ± 6	172 ± 30	70 ± 8	33 ± 7	37 ± 3
†Estrogen ⎡ 28	255 ± 35	14 ± 4	173 ± 22	68 ± 16	33 ± 11	35 ± 6
56	$225 \pm 30^{‡}$	13 ± 5	$130 \pm 23^{†}$	82 ± 20	$46 \pm 17§$	36 ± 7
⎣ 84	$256 \pm 41§$	12 ± 8	$169 \pm 27^{†}$	76 ± 18	37 ± 12	39 ± 6

VLDL = very low-density lipoproteins; IDL = intermediate density lipoprotein; LDL = low-density lipoprotein; HDL = high-density lipoprotein.

*Statistics are for each period versus the previous one.

†$p < .01$

‡$p < .02$

§$p < .05$

Reprinted with permission from D. Applebaum-Bowden et al. Estrogen reduces LDL cholesterol on a high cholesterol diet in post menopausal women. *Arteriosclerosis*, 2, p. 415A, 1982.

line following estrogen discontinuation. The significance of these changes remains unknown (and the physiological role of HTGL largely speculative). However, current theory would suggest that this enzyme may play a central role in the catabolism of HDL (Kuusi, Saarinen, & Nikkila, 1980; Shirai, Barnhart, & Jackson, 1981), perhaps via hydrolysis of the surface phospholipid on HDL, rendering the apolipoproteins A1 and A2 vulnerable to irreversible removal, thereby reducing the ability of HDL to scavange cholesterol from peripheral (e.g., arterial) tissues. Within this study subject group, for instance, a strong negative relationship existed after 28 days of estrogen therapy between their HDL_2 cholesterol levels and the activity of HTGL in their postheparin plasma: those with the highest HTGL activity on estrogen had the lowest HDL_2 cholesterol levels; those with the lowest HTGL activity had the highest HDL_2 cholesterol levels.

ANDROGEN SUPPLEMENTATION ON LIPROTEIN LIPIDS

But what of the effect of androgens on cholesterol levels in humans? These data are more difficult to obtain, but experience with androgenic anabolic steroids may lend insight. One such agent carefully studied in our laboratory is stanozolol, a 2, 3, nitrazine ring 17-alpha-methyl anabolic steroid. Because of some adverse effects noted in hyperlipidemic subjects taking the related anabolic steroid oxandrolone (Cheung, Albers, Wahl, & Hazzard, 1980), we were interested to examine the effects of stanozolol in postmenopausal osteoporotic women (Taggart et al., 1982), in whom this drug had previously been demonstrated to be associated with increased bone mineral content (Chesnut et al., 1983). Therefore, we studied 10 postmenopausal osteoporotic women during six weeks of therapy with stanozolol, 6 mg/day, a standard therapeutic dose (but far lower than the very large doses taken by power atheletes). During these studies, total cholesterol was not altered: this was accounted for by equal and offsetting changes in LDL and HDL. When examined as to mean percentage changes in these lipoprotein lipids (Figure 6.8), the ominous effects were clear: mean LDL levels increased 20%, and HDL decreased by nearly 50% (and the LDL/HDL ratio by nearly 60%), a uniform response among all 10 subjects. By one week after the androgen was discontinued, changes toward baseline were observed, but pretreatment levels were not clearly reached until 4 weeks later. Even more ominously, the HDL cholesterol levels were selectively reduced within the theoretically more antiatherogenic HDL_2 fraction, which declined an average of 85%. HDL_3 also declined, as did apo A-1 and, least of all, apo A-2.

Figure 6.8 Percent changes in mean plasma LDL-cholesterol (upward closed arrowhead), triglyceride (open circle), total cholesterol (closed circle), and HDL-cholesterol (open arrowhead) in ten postmenopausal osteoporotic women during (stippled area) and after treatment with stanozolol, 6 mg/per day.

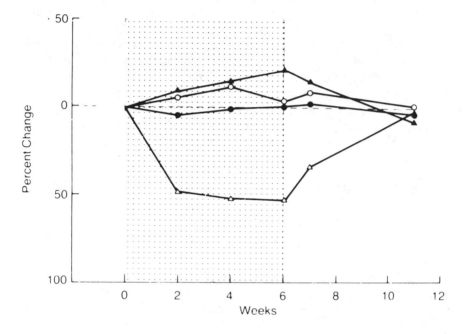

Reprinted with permission from H. M. Taggart et al. (1982). Reduction in high density lipoproteins by anabolic steroid (stanozolol) therapy for postmenopausal osteoporosis. *Metabolism, 31,* p. 1149.

As to the possible mechanism of this response, while HDL levels were declining, postheparin HTGL levels were increasing in these study subjects, by an average of nearly 300%. Moreover, daily measurements of HDL subfractions and postheparin HTGL early during stanozolol therapy in a separate group of subjects (4 women and 2 men) (Applebaum-Bowden, Haffner, & Hazzard, 1987) demonstrated a rise in HTGL within 24 hours, reaching a peak of greater than 250% of baseline by 4 days, whereas HDL_2 levels were not clearly diminished until 3 to 4 days of threatment (and HDL_3 did not change within the first 10 days of therapy). Finally, studies employing radiolabelled autologous HDL apolipoproteins disclosed a clear acceleration of HDL catabolism (notably HDL_3 and apolipoprotein A-2) during stanozolol treatment, consistent with an HTGL-mediated acceleration in HDL removal as the prime mechanism of this response (Haffner, Kushwana, Foster, Applebaum-Bowden, & Hazzard, 1983).

Figure 6.9 High-density lipoprotein cholesterol (HDL-C, circles) and low-density lipoprotein cholesterol (LDL-C, squares) levels during treatment of a postmenopausal woman with estrogen (ethinyl estradiol, 0.06 mg/per day), stanozolol (6 mg/per day), both, or neither. Solid bars indicate timing of HDL turnover studies. The subject had been on cyclic estrogen therapy for several years when these studies were initiated.

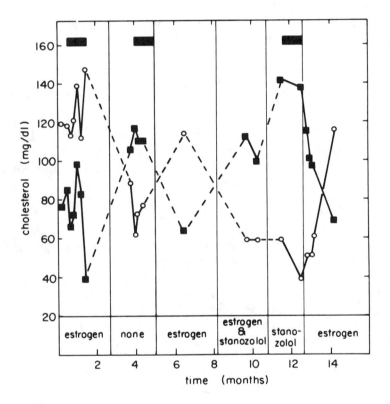

Reprinted with permission from W. R. Hazzard et al. (1984). Preliminary report: Kinetic studies on the modulation of high-density lipoprotein, apolipoprotein, and subfraction metabolism by sex steroids in a postmenopausal woman. *Metabolism, 33,* p. 780.

Additional studies in a single postmenopausal woman were particularly revealing (Figure 6.9) (Hazzard, Haffner, Kushwana, Applebaum-Bowden, & Foster, 1984). This subject was hypercholesterolemic when referred on estrogen therapy. However, this was attributable to *increased* concentrations of HDL, LDL actually being relatively depressed. Withdrawal of the estrogen was associated with an increase in LDL cholesterol and a decrease in HDL cholesterol, the reverse changes being evident when estrogen was reinstituted. When the combination of estrogen and stanozolol was given, her lipoprotein levels on both steroids were the same as they had been off both steroids. When stanozolol was given alone, LDL cholesterol levels became elevated, and HDL decreased. Finally, when she was placed back on estrogen, HDL levels were once again increased and LDL diminished. In serial studies in this subject of postheparin HTGL and radiolabelled HDL lipoprotein catabolism, the reciprocal effects of the two agents on HDL metabolism and HTGL were apparent: estrogen depressed postheparin HTGL and retarded HDL catabolism, whereas stanozolol increased post heparin HTGL and accelerated HDL catabolism.

SUMMARY

The studies previously described provide strong evidence to support the idea that steroids play a major role in the sex differtial in human longevity. This evidence comes from characterization of in vivo relationships, combined with their manipulation with exogenous steroids. The argument begins with the observations that cardiovascular disease is overwhelmingly the major cause of death, and the age-adjusted mortality rate is twice as high for males as it is for females. High cardiovascular disease risk is assocated with high LDL cholesterol levels, whereas low cardiovascular disease risk is associated with high HDL cholesterol levels. Finally, exogenous estrogens can raise HDL cholesterol and lower LDL cholesterol, whereas androgens have the opposite effect suggesting that males are naturally vulnerable because of their LDL/HDL cholesterol levels. Although the molecular basis for the effects of exogenous steroids has not been unequivocally demonstrated, several observations appear to be relevant. These include the fact that estrogen increases both LDL receptor activity and mRNA for the LDL receptor in rat and rabbit livers, respectively (Windler et al. 1980; Ma, Yamanoto, Goldstein, & Brown, 1986) as well as stimulates apolipoprotein A-1 and HDL synthesis in females (Schaefer et al., 1983). It remains to be seen whether estrogen also reduces HDL catabolism (Hazzard et al., 1984).

This scenario is likely to be overly simplistic as sex steroids influence a wide variety of biochemical parameters, many of which are relevant to atherogenesis. Moreover, multiple cultural and biobehavioral factors (perhaps also influenced by sex steroids) are also clearly important (Wingard, 1984). Thus, no single explanation is likely to completely explain the entirety of the almost universal biological phenomenon of greater female longevity.

REFERENCES

Applebaum-Bowden, D., Haffner, S. M., & Hazzard, W. R. (1987). The dyslipoproteinemia of anabolic steroid therapy: increase in hepatic triglyceride lipase precedes the decrease in high density lipoprotein$_2$ cholesterol. *Metabolism, 36,* 949–952.

Applebaum-Bowden, D., McLean, P., Steinmetz, A., Fontana, D., Matthys, C., Warnick, R., Cheung, M., & Albers, J. (1989). Lipoprotein, apolipoprotein, and lipolytic enzyme changes following estrogen administration in postmenopausal women. *J. Lipid Res., 30,* 1895–1906.

Bradley, D. D., Wingerd, J., Petit, D. B., Krauss, R. M., & Ramcharan, S. (1978). Serum high density lipoprotein cholesterol in women using oral contraceptives, estrogens, and progestins. *N Eng J Med, 299,* 17–20.

Chesnut, C. H. III, Ivey, J. L., Gruber, H. E., Matthew, M., Nelp, W. B., Sisom, K., & Baylink, D. J. (1983). Stanozolol in postmenopausal osteoporosis: therapeutic efficacy and possible mechanisms of action. *Metabolism, 32,* 571–580.

Cheung, M. C., Albers, J. J., Wahl, P. W., & Hazzard, W. R. (1980). High density lipoproteins during hypolipidemic therapy: a comparative study of four drugs. *Atherosclerosis, 35,* 215–228.

Eder, H. A. (1979). The rationale for measurement of HDL subclasses. In K. Lippel, (Ed.), Report of the High Density Lipoprotein Methodology Workshop, pp. 279–287. NIH Pub. N. 79–1661.

Haffner, S. M., Kushwaha, R. S., Foster, D. M., Applebaum-Bowden, D., & Hazzard, W. R. (1983). Studies on the metabolic mechanism of reduced high density lipoproteins during anabolic steroid therapy. *Metabolism, 32,* 413–420.

Hazzard, W. R. (1986). Biological basis of the sex differential in longevity. *J Am Geriatr Soc, 34,* 455–471.

Hazzard, W. R., Haffner, S. M., Kushwaha, R. S., Applebaum-Bowden, D., & Foster, D. M. (1984). Preliminary report: Kinetic studies on the modulation of high-density lipoprotein, apolipoprotein and subfraction metabolism by sex steriods in a postmenopausal woman. *Metabolism, 33,* 779–784.

Holden, C. (1983). Can smoking explain ultimate gender gap? *Science, 221,* 1034.

Kannel, W. B., & Brand, F. N. (1984). Cardiovascular risk factors in the elderly. In R. Andres, E. Bierman, & W. Hazzard, (Eds.), *Principles of geriatric medicine.* New York: McGraw-Hill.

Knopp, R. H., Walden, C. E., Wahl, P. W., Hoover, J. J., Warnick, G. R., Albers, J. J., Ogilvie, J. T., & Hazzard, W. R. (1981). Oral contraceptive and postmenopausal estrogen effects on lipoprotein triglyceride and cholesterol in an adult female population: relationships to estrogen and progestin potency. *J Clin Endrocrinol Metab, 53,* 1123–1132.

Kuusi, T., Saarinen, P., & Nikkila, E. A. (1980). Evidence for the role of hepatic endothelial lipase in the metabolism of plasma high density lipoprotein$_2$ in man. *Altherosclerosis, 36:*589–593.

Ma, P. T. S., Yamanoto, T., Goldstein, J. L., & Brown, M. S. (1986). Increased mRNA for low density lipoprotein receptor in livers of rabbits treated with 17α-ethinyl estradiol. *Proc Natl Acad Sci USA, 83*, 792–796.

Schaefer, E. J., Foster, D. M., Zech, L. A., Lindgren, F. T., Brewer, H. B., & Levy, R. I. (1983). The effects of estrogen administration on plasma lipoprotein metabolism in premenopausal females. *J Clin Endocrinol Metab, 57*, 262–267.

Shirai, K., Barnhart, R. L., & Jackson, R. L. (1981). Hydrolysis of human plasma high density lipoprotein$_2$ phospholipids and triglycerides by hepatic lipase. *Biochem Biophys Res Commun, 100*, 591–599.

Sullivan, J. L. (1983). The sex differential in ischemic heart disease. *Perspectives in Biology and Medicine, 26*, 657–671.

Taggart, H. M., Applebaum-Bowden, D., Haffner, S., Warnick, G. R., Cheung, M. C., Albers, J. J., Chesnut, C. H. III, & Hazzard, W. R. (1982). Reduction in high density lipoproteins by anabolic steroid (stanozolol) therapy for postmenopausal osteoporosis. *Metabolism, 31*, 1147–1152.

Wahl, P., Walden, C., Knopp, R., Hoover, J., Wallace, R., Heiss, G., & Rifkind, B. (1983). Effect of estrogen/progestin potency on lipid/lipoprotein cholesterol. *N Eng J Med, 308*, 862–867.

Wallace, R. B., Hoover, J., Barrett-Connor, E., Rifkind, B. M., Hunninghake, D. B., Mackenthun, A., & Heiss, G. (1979). Altered plasma lipid and liporotein levels associated with oral contraceptive and oestrogen use. *Lancet, II*, 111–115.

Windler, E. E. T., Kovanen, P. T., Chao, Y., Brown, M. S., Havel, R. J., & Goldstein, J. L. (1980). The estradiol-stimulated lipoprotein receptor of rat liver: a binding site that mediates the uptake of rat lipoproteins containing apoproteins B and E. *J Biol Chem, 255*, 10464–10471.

Wingard, D. L. (1984). The sex differential in morbidity, mortality and lifestyle. *Ann Rev Pub Health, 5*, 433–458.

7 A Possible Role for the Immune System in the Gender-Longevity Differential

Marc E. Weksler

The capacity of the female of various mammalian species, including man, to outperform the male when measured in terms of immune responsiveness has been documented many times.

Eidinger and Garrett, 1972

This statement offers a possible mechanism to explain the longer life span of women in our society. One could formulate the hypothesis that the greater immunological vigor of women provides them with greater resistance to disease and thereby with longer life. The scientific literature contains evidence that supports the primary supposition, that is, that females of several species have greater immune reactivity than males. Acceptance of this hypothesis is limited, to a far greater extent, by the paucity of evidence that immune vigor is directly related to life span.

The primary goal of this brief review is to bring together data relevant to this hypothesis. The reader will find that there is considerable evidence that gender is an important determinant of immune reactivity. However, it is perfectly clear that both gender and age affect the immune response, and that interrelations among gender, immunity, and age are extremely complex.

The age of an animal has an important influence on the effect of gender on the immune response. The most obvious reason for this is the age-associated changes in gonadal function resulting in altered levels of circulating sex hormones. Surprisingly, only one study exists (Belisle & Strausser, 1981) comparing animals of different sexes at various times during their life span. These authors emphasize the importance of life span studies by the different response to phytohemagglutinin (PHA) or concanavalin A (Con A) of lymphocytes

Supported in part by USPHS grant P01 AG00541.

from male and female mice between the ages of 2, 14, and 24 months. The proliferative response of T lymphocytes (T cells) from female animals was greater between 2 and 14 months, but this difference was reversed when 24-month-old mice were compared. The reason for this change was the more rapid decline with age in the proliferative response of T cells from female mice compared to male mice.

It is possible that, in addition to extrinsic influences of gender on the immune system brought about by sex hormones, the function of lymphocytes or accessory cells from males or females of the same species differs due to factors intrinsic to the cells. Obviously, these cells differ in their chromosomal complement in the sense that cells from males have an X- and a Y-chromosome whereas cells from females have two X-chromosomes, but the function of immune cells taken from male or female donors and transferred into castrated, syngeneic animals has not been studied. Whatever the reality of an intrinsic effect of gender on the cells of the immune system, there is much evidence that the predominant effect results from the influence of sex hormones on immune activity.

Before accepting the evidence that females of a species have greater immune reactivity than males of the same species, the reader should keep in mind that: (a) most studies have been limited to a few strains or species; (b) significant effects of gender on immunity may be present at one age and not seen, or reversed, at other ages; and (c) reports exist in which no significant effect of gender on immune function has been found (Kniker, Anderson, McBryde, Roumiantzeff, & Lesourd, 1984).

There is a consensus that young sexually mature female mice (2 to 3 months of age) produce more antibody following immunization with either thymic-dependent or thymic-independent antigens than do male mice of the same age. Thus, in the outbred Swiss albino mice studied by Terres, Morrison, & Habicht (1968), both the primary and secondary responses to bovine serum albumin were significantly greater in female than in male mice. In the primary immune response, female mice produced specific antibody more rapidly after immunization, had a peak level of serum antibody 2 to 4 times greater than that of male mice, and had detectable specific antibody for a longer time following immunization. Female mice had an even greater response relative to males in the secondary response. This did not appear to result from a difference in the catabolism of antibody as there was no significant difference in the capacity of male and female mice to degrade antigen–antibody complexes.

In another study, Eidinger and Garrett (1972) reported that female inbred mice immunized with either a thymus-dependent (xenogeneic erythrocytes) or a thymus-independent (polyvinyl-pyrrolidone) antigen produced more IgM antibody during the primary response, and more IgG antibody during the secondary response, than did male mice of the same strain and age. Castration of the male mice enhanced their immune response, suggesting an extrinsic effect of the gonads on the immune system.

Few studies have searched for the cellular basis for the increased antibody response of female mice. In one study, the increased serum antibody concentration was found to be associated with an increased number of splenic antigen-specific plaque-forming cells. (Krzych, Thurman, Goldstein, Bressler, & Strausser, 1979). Thus, the number of antisheep erythrocytes and antilipopolysaccharide plaque-forming cells was higher in female mice immunized in vivo with these antigens. Weinstein, Ran, and Segal, (1984) provided evidence that accessory cells from female mice were more efficient in presenting antigen than were accessory cells from male animals. The reports that phagocytosis is greater in female than in male animals may be relevant to antigen processing by accessory cells. This difference in phagocytic capacity appears to be under estrogenic control. Also of interest was the report that neonatal thymectomy abolished sex differences in the immune response (Terres et al, 1968). Whether gender also influences the function of B or T lymphocytes has not been established.

Autoantibodies and autoimmune disease are more common in females of many animal species and in humans (Rowley, Buchanan, & Mackay, 1968). The frequency of benign monoclonal antibodies in mice following neonatal thymectomy is also greater in female than male animals (Radl, DeGlopper, Vandenberg, & VanZwietin, 1980). It is not certain whether such abnormalities should be considered immune "vigor" or, more likely immune dysregulation.

There is convincing evidence that castration of male animals and estrogen therapy of autoimmune mice favors the development of disease, while the administration of androgens suppresses the expression of the disease (Weinstein et al., 1984). Testosterone is also known to affect the size of the thymus gland, a central organ of immune development. The thymus is larger in females than in males and orchiectomy, but not ovariectomy, results in thymic hypertrophy and a delay in thymic involution.

The more frequent and earlier expression of autoantibodies in females than males suggests a lesser degree of self-tolerance. The ability of male and female mice to be rendered tolerant to foreign antigens has not been systematically studied, but in the only study found in the literature that compares the influence of gender on the sensitivity to tolerance induction, female mice were more difficult to render tolerant than male mice. Thus, Dresser (1962) showed that "high dose" tolerance to bovine gamma globulin was more difficult to establish in female than in male mice. There is also evidence that cell-mediated immunity is more vigorous in female inbred mice. Congeneic skin grafts were rejected by more female mice (55%) than by male mice (28%) (Graff, Lappe, & Snell, 1969). Furthermore, rejection was significantly more rapid in the females, as median graft survival was 16 days in female recipients, compared to 21 days in male recipients.

The capacity of T cells from male or female mice to proliferate in vitro has been studied by a number of investigators. There seems to be reasonable concordance in their results. First of all, the greatest difference in the cellular responses between males and females seems to occur when spleen cell reactions are measured. In fact, spleen cells, but not lymph node cells or thymocytes, from female mice incorporated more tritiated thymidine than spleen cells from male mice when cultured with Con A or lipopolysaccharide (Krzych et al., 1979).

The influence of sex hormones on the proliferation of murine spleen cells in the allogeneic mixed lymphocyte reaction (MLR) was studied by Weinstein et al. (1984). In this study, lymphocytes from either female or male mice that have a genetic defect that prevents the production or response to testosterone were more reactive than lymphocytes from normal male mice. Furthermore, when testosterone-deficient mice were given estrogen their response to allogeneic cells increased further. Greater in vitro proliferative response of spleen cells from female mice was also observed following in vivo immunization with protein antigens. Lymphocytes from female mice incorporated more thymidine than did lymphocytes from male mice or female mice treated with testosterone. In these studies, accessory cells from female mice were more efficient in initiating a secondary response in vitro than cells from male mice. Finally, castration of male mice enhanced, and treatment of female mice with androgen reduced, the efficiency of antigen presentation.

In virtually all the studies that have compared the immune response of male and female animals, sexually mature young animals have been examined. Most mice have been studied between 2 and 3 months of age. These animals have completed less than 15% of their life span. The difficulty in generalizing from studies of such young animals is illustrated by the only study that measured the proliferative response of BALB/c splenic cells from mice 2, 6, 9, 12, 14, and 24 months of age (Belisle & Strausser, 1981). In this study, the response of B lymphocytes from females to lipopolysaccharide was greater than that of B cells from males between the ages of 2 and 24 months. However, although the response to PHA and Con A was greater in females than males between 2 and 14 months of age, at 24 months of age the response was greater in males than females. Furthermore, in another substrain (BALB/cAnNCrlBr) tested, no significant sex differences in these responses were observed.

Most of the studies comparing immune responses in male and female animals have employed mice. In none of these studies has the life span of the female and male animals been reported. Where life span of male and female mice have been compared, immune function has not been reported with respect to the sex of the animals measured. In one study, (Gordon, Bruckner-Kardoss, & Wostmann, 1966) male mice maintained in a conventional environment had a significantly shorter life span than females. When mice of the same strain were maintained in a germ-free environment, both male and female mice lived longer, with the males having a significantly longer life span than females. The reason for these changes in life span with respect to survival of male and female mice is not clear, but one can speculate that when animals are exposed to a conventional environment the greater immune response of female mice may contribute to their longer life. In the absence of bacterial stress, the difference in immune reactivity becomes less important and other factors favor the survival of the male animals.

Few studies that have directly addressed the relationship between immune activity and survival have been performed in man. Studies have measured immune function in older persons and correlated the immune activity of persons who died with those who survived a specified period of time. The data suggest that old subjects with better preserved immune function have longer survival. In these studies, groups of old humans were studied with respect to delayed-type cutaneous reactivity (Roberts-Thomson, Wittingham, Youngchaiyud, & Mackay, 1974), with respect to the presence of serum autoantibodies (Mackay, 1972), and with respect to altered suppressor cell activity (Hallgren & Yunis, 1980). The old persons were then followed for two years and their survival was correlated with immunological abnormalities. The presence of immune abnormalities was associated with shortened survival. These studies did not report an association with the gender of the subjects. There are several inherent problems in such studies. The most important is the difficulty in distinguishing between immune deficiency that leads to disease and death, and immune deficiency that results from preexisting, subclinical disease that leads to the death of the subject. Finally, it is not clear whether relative immune deficiency is correlated with gender.

SUMMARY

Young female animals produce more autoantibodies, monoclonal immunoglobulins, and more specific antibody following immunization with foreign antigens. Young female animals reject skin grafts more actively and have greater T lymphocyte proliferative responses than do T cells from young male animals. It is uncertain whether these early differences in immune responses between the sexes persist throughout the life span or whether these immunological differences lead to biological "advantage" and longer life of female animals. Careful studies correlating immunological activity of male and female mice with their survival would permit an association of sex, immune reactivity, and life span to be made. Only then could one really test the hypothesis that immune reactivity contributes to life span. Until such studies are completed, it will be impossible to do more than speculate about an association among the heightened immune activity of female animals, the longer survival of elderly humans with better preserved immune function, and the longer life span of women in our society.

REFERENCES

Belisle, E. H., & Strausser, H. R. (1981). Sex-related immunocompetence of BALB/c mice. *Developmental and Comparative Immunology, 5,* 661–670.

Dresser, D. W. (1962). Specific inhibition of antibody production. *Immunology, 5,* 161–168.

Eidinger, D., & Garrett, T. J. (1972). Studies on the regulation effects of the sex hormones on antibody formation and stem cell differentiation. *J. of Experimental Medicine, 13,* 1098–1116.

Gordon, H. A., Bruckner-Kardoss, E., & Wostmann, B. S. (1966). Aging in germ-free mice: Life tables and lesions observed at natural death. *Journal of Gerontology, 21,* 380–387.

Graff, R. J., Lappe, M. A., & Snell, G. D. (1969). The influence of the gonads and adrenal glands on the immune response to skin grafts. *Transplantation, 7,* 105–111.

Hallgren, H. M., & Yunis, E. J. (1981). Immune function, immune regulation, and survival in an aging human population. In D. Segre & L. Smith (Eds.), *Immunological aspects of aging* (pp. 281–293). New York: Marcel Dekker.

Kniker, W. T., Anderson, C. T., McBryde, J. L., Roumiantzeff, M., & Lesourd, B. (1984). Multitest CMI for standarized measurement of delayed cutaneous hypersensitivity and cell-mediated immunity. Normal values and proposed scoring system for healthy adults in the U.S.A. *Annals of Allergy, 52,* 75–82.

Krzych, U, Thuman, G. B., Goldstein, A. L., Bressler, J. P., & Strausser, H. R. (1979). Sex-related immunocompetence of BALB/c mice. *Journal of Immunology, 123,* 2568–2574.

Mackay, I. R. (1972). Aging and immunological function in man. *Gerontologia, 18,* 285–304.

Radl, J., DeGlopper, E., Vandenberg, P., & VanZwieten, M. J. (1980). Idiopathic paraproteinemia. *Journal of Immunology, 125,* 31–35.

Roberts-Thomson, I. C., Wittingham, S., Youngchaiyud, D., & Mackay, I. R. (1974). Aging, immune response and mortality. *Lancet, II,* 368–370.

Rowley, M. J., Buchanan, H., & Mackay, I. R. (1968). Reciprocal changes with age in antibody to extrinsic and intrinsic antigens. *Lancet, II,* 24–26.

Terres, G., Morrison, S. L., & Habicht, G. S. (1968). A quantitative difference in the immune response between male and female mice. *Proceedings of the Society for Experimental Biology and Medicine, 127,* 664–667.

Weinstein, Y., Ran, S., & Segal, S. (1984). Sex-associated differences in the regulation of immune responses controlled by the MHC of the mouse. *Journal of Immunology, 132,* 656–661.

III THE IMPACT OF SOCIAL ROLES ON HEALTH AND HEALTH CARE USE

8 Multiple Roles for Middle-Aged Women and their Impact on Health

Sonja M. McKinlay
Randi S. Triant
John B. McKinlay
Donald J. Brambilla
Matthew Ferdock

Middle-aged women, between about 40 and 60 years of age, are a subgroup of the population about whom surprisingly little is known. Despite the fact that middle-aged women are one of the fastest growing subgroups (U.S. Department of Labor, 1985), most available information concerning these women has been obtained indirectly through studies of the elderly and of men. For example, it is well-established that women in this age-range are frequently primary, informal caregivers to ailing or frail elderly parents (or parents-in-law) (Brody, 1981; McKinlay & Tennstedt, 1986). They are also the most important source of support for men recovering from heart attacks, and may play an important role in determining a man's risk of heart disease (Croog & Levine, 1977; Haynes & Feinleib, 1980).

These important support roles have been documented, albeit from indirect and fragmented studies. Other important roles, such as worker, have been largely overlooked. Moreover, the impact of these roles, particularly the support roles, on women's own health, has been largely ignored. The few studies of work and health that included women largely examined the effect that work has on their family or marital relationships. Much less attention has been paid to the effect of employment on women's health and well-being. Reviewing research studies in the late 1970s, Welch and Booth (1977) emphasized the need for longitudinal studies in this area. Yet, little over a decade later, there is still a paucity of longitudinal research focusing on the contribution of

This investigation is supported by National Institute of Aging Grant No. AG03111 work to the health status of women. This continued dearth of research is especially notable given women's increased labor force participation throughout the eighties (U.S. Department of Labor, 1985).

Recently, debate has begun to focus on whether multiple roles (career plus family demands) are deleterious to a woman's overall health (Rice & Cugliani, 1979; Verbrugge, 1983). Women have increasingly taken on the role of worker in addition to that of spouse, mother, and informal caregiver (Verbrugge, 1983). Support for the increased participation of women in the labor force was met with equally vocal criticism. Critics claimed that women were now forced to deal not only with the demands of a job, but also had the double burden of continued responsibility for household management and all child care needs (Verbrugge, 1983).

Lewin-Epstein (1986) in an extensive review of multiple-role research, identifies two theoretical perspectives for explaining the relationship between employment and health. The nurturant-role viewpoint suggests that the addition of demanding roles (e.g., worker) to the traditional nurturing role of women results in a greater disposition towards poor health and increased rates of morbidity due to role overload and role strain (Gove & Huges, 1979; Gove & Tudor, 1973; Woods & Hulka, 1979). The fixed-role obligations perspective suggests that health behavior may be related to time constraints resulting from role obligations (Nathanson, 1975, 1980). Therefore, "women who occupy work roles in addition to familial roles will be less likely to adopt the sick role and engage in illness behavior" simply because they are too busy fulfilling their fixed roles to be sick (Lewin-Epstein, 1986, p. 1172).

Thus, some studies have suggested that the addition of job responsibilities may lead to increased stress, fatigue, Type-A behavior patterns and coronary heart disease (Gove & Tudor, 1973; Haynes & Feinleib, 1980; Haynes, Feinleib, & Levine, 1978; Meisenhelder, 1986; Nathanson, 1975). However, other studies have found that the increased social interaction, enhanced organization skills and the prestige that a job gives have a positive effect on the overall health of women (Jennings, Mazaik, & McKinlay, 1984; Marcus & Seeman, 1981; Meisenhelder, 1986; Mostow & Newberry, 1975; Nathanson, 1980; Verbrugge, 1983; Verbrugge, 1985; Welch & Booth, 1977).

Prior research, because of small sample sizes, short study duration, or inherent biases has failed to indicate more definitely whether work is indeed a boon or a bane (Cochrane & Stope-Roe, 1981; Gove & Geerken, 1977; Grossman, 1977; Hauensten, Kasl & Harburg, 1977; Howell, 1973; Lewin-Epstein, 1986; Meisenhelder, 1986; Mostow & Newberry, 1975; Parry, 1986; Verbrugge, 1983; Waldron, Herold,

Donn & Staum, 1982). Waldron (1978, p. 435) summed up the situation when they wrote "the available data do not provide an adequate basis for estimating the overall effects of employment on women's health in the contemporary United States."

The purpose of this chapter is to address prior research inadequacies by examining prospective data gathered over nearly four years on a randomly selected cohort of approximately 2,500 middle-aged women. Specifically, this chapter will present empirical findings on four important topics:

1. The relationship of employment status changes to women's health and functioning.
2. The distribution of three different nurturing or support roles (spouse, mother, caregiver) in relation to work status.
3, The stress impact of these roles.
4. The combined effect of multiple roles and resulting stress on concurrent health status.

METHODS

Sample

Analyses to address the first topic are based on data collected from a randomly sampled cohort of about 2,000 women from Massachusetts initially aged 45 to 55, participating in a five-year prospective study of women approaching and experiencing the menopause.[1] Telephone interviews of approximately 30 minutes' duration were conducted with the cohort once every nine months. A wide variety of data were collected at baseline (T_0) and five follow-up interviews (T_1–T_5); only information on employment history, education, age, health, insurance, menopausal status, use of prescription drugs, psychological symptoms, physical symptoms, and chronic conditions are reported here. Complete follow-up information on these variables are available for nearly 2,000 of the originally eligible cohort.

For analysis of the remaining three topics, only those completing a supplemental interview on aspects of life-style at the fourth and fifth interviews were included ($n=1,599$). These supplemental interviews contained questions on care of parents (or parents-in-law). The subgroup represents a random two-thirds sample of the original cohort. A random one-third received the supplement at T_4, another random

[1]Refer to McKinlay et al., 1987 for more detailed description of this study.

one-third received it at T_5. These supplemental data (T_4 or T_5) were combined with concurrently collected data from the core interview on employment, stress, household composition, and health to form a cross-sectional data set for analysis.

It should be noted that, for all analyses, drop-out of cohort members (from death, refusal, or loss to follow-up) was negligible (less than 10% through all follow-up contacts). Further, because only premenopausal women were selected for the cohort, the sample has a positively skewed age distribution, is somewhat better educated than the general population of women the same age, and report a lower rate of cigarette smoking, consistent with their higher socioeconomic and premenopausal status (McKinlay, Bifano, & McKinlay, 1985).

Variables

Using the most reliable methodologies currently available, self-report data were obtained on each respondent's health status as well as on sociodemographic circumstances. Measures of *health status* included physical and psychological symptoms, chronic conditions, self-assessed health, and the Center for Epidemiological Studies Depression-Scale (CES-D) depression score. Symptoms, self-assessed health and the CES-D scale were measured at each interval while new chronic conditions were cumulated from T_0 (omitting those mentioned at T_0) to T_5. Respondents were asked to indicate whether any of several common symptoms had been experienced in the past two weeks. Eliminating symptoms that relate to either menstruation or menopause (hot flashes/flushes, cold sweats, and menstrual problems), the remaining symptoms were subdivided somewhat arbitrarily into two groups: common physical symptoms, including diarrhea and/or constipation, persistent cough, upset stomach, backaches, headaches, sore throat, and aches/stiffness in the joints; and those that appear primarily psychological in origin, such as dizzy spells, lack of energy, irritability, feeling blue or depressed, shortness of breath, trouble sleeping, and loss of appetite. Self-assessed health in relation to one's peers (worse, same, better) is well known as a valid measure of current overall health status (Maddox, 1964). The Center for Epidemiological Studies in Depression Scale (Radloff, 1977) is one of the few valid, reliable measures of depression applicable in population-based investigations.

Menopausal status was determined for each respondent at each interval based on a combination of questions on current menstrual status and change in the last nine months. Women were considered *premenopausal* if they reported regular menses in the last three months.

Women were classified as *perimenopausal* if menses had been reported in the last twelve months, but with periods of amenorrhea and/or changes in regularity or flow. This definition is consistent with prior research (Jaszmann, 1969; Magursky, Mesko, Sokolik, 1975; Treloar, 1974). Women were considered to be naturally *post-menopausal* if no menses were reported for twelve months, in the absence of surgery that would terminate menstruation. Twelve months of amenorrhea is the widely accepted definition used in European studies since the 1950s (see, for example, Magursky, Mesko, & Sokolik, 1975) and is recommended by Treloar (1974) on the basis of his prospective study of normal menstrual patterns. *Surgical menopause* was considered to have occurred if menses were surgically stopped; *either* a hysterectomy (with or without removal of the ovaries) *or* a bilateral oopherectomy (occurring in none of the cohort as of T_5).

Sociodemographic information, determined at baseline, included age and education. Household income was not considered as an indicator of socioeconomic status for this analysis because a large subgroup (14%) failed to provided this information. Many of these women reported that they did not know what their husbands earned. Educational status (years of education, in three categories), which is known to be strongly associated with both per capita income and occupational status, was therefore chosen as a reasonable indicator of socioeconomic status for this analysis. Because presence or absence of health insurance may affect utilization of health services and hence affect diagnosis of health conditions, insurance status (measured at each time point) was also considered.

Employment status was ascertained at each interval. Five categories were established to determine a respondent's employment change between T_0 and T_5. Women were considered employed throughout (EE) if they were employed at each followup. Those women who were employed at T_0 but became unemployed at some point during the next five follow-ups (and remained unemployed) were classified as employed/unemployed (EU). Those women who were unemployed at T_0 but became employed at some point during the next five followups and remained employed were classified as unemployed/employed (UE). Women who were intermittently employed (i.e., had changed their employment status more than once) were considered in the intermittent category (IN). Finally, women were considered unemployed throughout (UU) if they had remained unemployed or were not in the labor force from T_0 to T_5.

Finally, to address the third and fourth topics, *stress* was measured as the answer to the question "In the past nine months has anyone close to you caused you any special worry?" If an affirmative answer was given, the person (or persons) were identified (e.g., husband, daughter, parent, boss).

Analytic Approach

The analyses addressing the relationship between employment changes and health are based on means and net difference scores. The frequency of psychological symptoms and physical symptoms reported at baseline (T_0) were subtracted from respective frequencies at T_5 (i.e., T_5-T_0). Similarly, the net change in those reporting health worse than their peers, or restriction in usual activity, was calculated. Mean differences or percentage changes were then calculated and tested for significant departures from zero in each employment change category controlling in turn: education, age, insurance, and menopausal status at the last interview. Student's t-tests (two-tailed, $p=.01$) were performed. The mean frequency of new chronic conditions was calculated from the cumulative number of new conditions diagnosed in the prior nine months, as reported in the five interviews. These mean frequencies were plotted (with 99% confidence intervals) for each employment change category controlling in turn: education, age, insurance, and menopausal status at the last interview. In as much as this range of scores overlapped (or failed to overlap) significant differences were determined.

The primary analytic approach employed in the cross-sectional data set used to address the remaining three topics was a stepwise fisherian discriminant, using linear regression and dichotomous dependent variables measuring health. Independent variables were added in sets, with the variables significant at the 0.01 level remaining fixed in the discriminant for the addition of the next set. In building the discriminants, the sociodemographic variables were added first, followed by the role indicators and finally the stress indicators.

RESULTS

Employment Change and Health

The distribution of the five employment change categories for the cohort is presented in Table 8.1. A very small proportion (just over 10%) of this middle-aged cohort remained unemployed or outside the labor force for the four years of observation. A larger proportion (nearly 15%) were intermittently employed and about the same proportion

Table 8.1 Distribution of Employment Change Over Four Years for 1944 Women Aged 45 to 55 at Baseline

Employment Change	Percent Distribution
Employed Throughout (EE)	61.1
Employed/Unemployed (EU)	6.7
Unemployed/Employed (UE)	7.2
Intermittently Employed (IN)	14.3
Unemployed Throughout (UU)	10.7
TOTAL (100%)	1944

either entered or left the employed sector in the same period, and in equivalent numbers. In other words, nearly 30% were variably in the work force during a four-year period, while 60% were constantly employed.

When these employment changes are related to health-status changes in the same period, the only significant associations are with physical and psychological symptoms. Table 8.2 indicates clearly, that, despite aging of the cohort and transitions through menopause for about half the women, patterns of employment are related to subsequent symptom reporting. Those women who stayed employed throughout, who were intermittently employed, or who became employed showed a significant decrease in the reported physical and psychological symptoms over the four years of observation. *No change*

Table 8.2 Employment Status and Changes in Physical and Psychological Symptoms

Employment change	T_0 levels		Significant decrease	No change
EE	Phys	= 1.4	Both	
	Psych	= 1.4		
EU	Phys	= 1.5		Both
	Psych	= 1.5		
IN	Phys	= 1.6	Both	
	Psych	= 1.6		
UE	Phys	= 1.4	Psychological	
	Psych	= 1.5		
UU	Phys	= 1.2		Both
	Psych	= 1.2		

EE, employed throughout; EU, employed/unemployed; IN, intermittently employed; UE, unemployed/employed; UU, unemployed throughout.

in either physical or psychological symptoms was found for those women who either became unemployed at some point or remained unemployed throughout the five years.

With respect to self-assessed health, there was no marked change in the four year period with some deterioration reported (p < 0.05) for only the employed/unemployed, intermittently employed, or continuously unemployed groups. No change was evident for those who remained or became employed. The number of new chronic conditions was slightly higher for women becoming unemployed, suggesting that some women may leave the labor force for health reasons, but the effect is not statistically significant. Although these results suggest a healthy worker effect (those with no change most likely to have become or remain employed), it does not produce significant differences ($p \leq 0.01$) and is not consistent with the above findings on acute symptoms.

When investigated, the effects of age, education, health insurance status at baseline, and menopause status at last contact on the above-mentioned relationships were negligible.

This analysis clearly indicates that women do not leave the work force primarily for health reasons. Moreover, the evidence suggests that employment has a positive impact on perceived health (is accompanied by a significant *decrease* in symptoms and no change in other measures of perceived health), which is contradictory to the changes that could be expected with aging and menopause. No increase in symptomatology was observed in the variably employed or unemployed groups.

Distribution of Roles

The second issue addressed by this analysis involves the estimation of the number and types of roles assumed by middle-aged women. The distribution of nurturing roles for women in this sample is summarized in Table 8.3. The majority (over 80%) of the total sample clearly reported performing at least two of the four roles considered (percentages in parentheses in Table 8.3). Nearly 50% performed at least three, and almost 10% of the sample performed all four roles (spouse, parent, worker, and caregiver for an elderly parent).

Working women comprise nearly three-quarters of the sample as reported at the last two contacts. In all cases working is an additional, not a substitute role. Further analysis of this sample of women aged 48 to 58 indicates that over 50% have both husband and children living at home and 80% of these women have additional roles (work and/or caregiver). The Chi-square test for independence of work from nurtur-

Table 8.3 The Distribution of Three Nurturing Roles[a], by Employment Status, for 1,595 Women[b]

Number of Nurturing roles	Working for pay	
	No	Yes
None	6.2 (1.7)[c]	11.6 (8.5)
One	30.5 (8.0)	29.6 (21.8)
Two	49.2 (13.0)	46.0 (34.0)
Three	14.1 (3.6)	12.8 (9.4)
Total (100%)	419 (26.3)	1,176 (73.7)

[a] The nurturing roles are: spouse, parent, caregiver.
[b] χ^2 test for independence of work from nurturing roles: $\chi^2_3 = 9.83$; $0.05 < p < 0.01$.
[c] The percentages in parentheses are of the total sample of 1595 women.

ing roles (Table 8.3) was significant only at the 0.05 level and primarily reflects the fact that more unmarried women were working, without other roles.

The Association of Stress with Three Nurturing Roles

Presence of each of the roles (spouse, parent, caregiver, and worker) was then related to whether or not individuals identified these roles as sources of stress. Table 8.4 presents the percentage identifying husbands as a source of stress, by whether or not a husband is present at home. Only about 5% of the sample reported husbands as a source of stress. The small percentage reporting this source of stress, even though there is no husband at home, includes women recently divorced or separated from their spouse.

Table 8.4 Percentage for Whom Husbands Are a Source of Stress, by Whether or Not a Husband Is at Home

Husband's status	Distribution of Husband's status		Percentage causing stress
	Number	Percentage	
Not at Home	388	24.3	3.6
At Home	1,208	75.7	6.3
Total	1,596	100.0	5.6

Table 8.5 Percentage for Whom Children Are a Source of Stress, by Whether or Not Children Are at Home

Status of children[a]	Distribution of children status		Percentage causing stress
	Number	Percentage	
Child(ren) not at home	516	32.4	8.5
Child(ren) at home	970	60.9	20.3
Child(ren) just arrived back home	106	6.7	23.6
Total	1,592	100.0	16.7

[a]Since prior interview.

Given the age-range of the sample, the respondents were likely to have adolescent or adult children about to leave home or who had recently left. The role of parent (children at home) was therefore divided into three categories: those with no children at home for more than nine months (including those without children and those whose children had left home); those who had children at home for more than nine months; and those who had no children at home nine months ago and had at least one child returning home in the last nine months. As indicated in Table 8.5 having children return home was the parent role most closely related to reported stress (nearly 24% reported stress from this situation). Still having children at home was seen as nearly as stressful (20% reported stress). The small percentage reporting stress among those with no children at home indicates a real reduction in stress with children leaving home, as only about one-fifth of this group reported having no children at all.

Finally, Table 8.6 relates caring for a parent (or parent-in-law) to identification of a parent as a source of stress. A quarter of the sample reported caring for a parent. Half of these women who provided parent care reported that a parent caused stress. There is remarkably little difference in the rate of stress reported when the parent is living with the respondent as compared with nonresidential care situations. Although no estimate of the proportion of respondents with no parent or parent-in-law alive is available from this study, it is likely to be small (probably less than 10%) given available estimates of life expectancy.

A boss or co-worker was almost never cited as a source of worry. Because no direct question was asked concerning the stress of the work situation itself, it was not possible to investigate the stress of the work role further. Moreover, the wording of the question may have resulted

Table 8.6 Percentage for Whom Parents (in-law) Are a Source of Stress, by Whether or Not Care is Provided

Provision of care	Distribution of care provision		Percentage causing stress
	Number	Percentage	
No care provided (or no parents)	1,196	75.0	13.0
Care provided to parent outside R's home	344	21.6	49.1
Care provided to parent in R's home	55	3.4	52.7
Total	1,595	100.0	22.2

in underreporting of work-related stress. Certainly, it is clear from these data that the three nurturing roles were sources of stress. At least in this study, the lack of negative health perception among working women (Jennings, Mazaik, & McKinlay, 1984) provides some indirect evidence that work was not a major source of stress for these women. The limitation of the stress question asked precludes direct evidence of work stress.

The Combined Effect of Roles and Stress on Health

Given the distribution of roles and their relationship to reported stress, these variables were then considered as potential discriminators of negative health outcomes controlling for age and education (as a measure of socioeconomic status).

Table 8.7 summarizes the best discriminant models estimated for each of six health outcomes considered in this chapter. Two distinct patterns are evident, each for three of the outcomes.

Self-assessed health, restricted activity, and new chronic conditions are related primarily to employment status and secondarily to stress caused by a spouse. As expected from the initial analyses, working women are less likely to report worse health, restricted activity days, or new chronic conditions, all measures of more chronic health status. This would appear to indicate a healthy worker effect. However, the presence of a husband as a source of stress in two of the discriminants required more detailed investigation. Further examination revealed that reporting of worse health did not vary for working women, by whether or not a spouse caused worry. However, among women who were not employed, those reporting worse health were most often those

Table 8.7 Discriminant Models for Five Health Outcomes

Discriminant variables	Health Outcomes[a]					
	Self-assessed health	Restricted activity days	Chronic conditions	Physical symptoms	Psychological symptoms	CES-D score[b]
Sociodemographic characteristics	Education	—	—	Education	Education	(Education)[b]
Roles	Work (Spouse)	Work	(Work)	Caregiver	Caregiver	Caregiver (Work) (Spouse)
Source of Stress	Husband	(Husband)	—	Husband child(ren)	Husband child(ren)	Husband child(ren)

[a]The health outcomes were dichotomized for discriminant analyses as follows: Self-assessed health worse = 1 (same/better = 0); 2+ Physical symptoms = 1 (one or none = 0); 2+ Psychological symptoms = 1 (one or none = 0); 1+ Restricted activity days = 1 (none = 0); CES-D score $\geq$ 16 = 1 ($<$ 16 = 0); and 1+ new chronic conditions = 1 (none = 0).
[b]Parentheses indicate significance of the coefficient at the 0.05 level only. All others are significant at the 0.01 level.

whose husbands were a source of stress. Despite small numbers in some groups, there is clear evidence among nonworking women that identification of a husband as a source of stress has additive effects on the percentage reporting worse health. This additive effect is not evident for working women. For restricted activity days, the association is reversed, with an effect of stress from a spouse only apparent for working women.

The pattern is somewhat different for the remaining three outcomes that are measures of acute health status. The dominant role afffecting health is that of caregiver. Yet, the stress caused by this role does not add significantly to the model (possibly because the level of stress associated with this role is so high—see Table 8.6). Instead, additional negative effects on health are contributed by stress from a spouse and children.

When the joint impact on these outcomes of the caregiver roles and stress caused by husband and/or children is investigated further, a clear pattern emerges in the varying rates of negative effects (Table 8.8).

Among those women not caring for a parent (or parent-in-law), stress from children or a spouse markedly increases the rates of negative health outcomes for all three measures considered. The increase is greater in the presence of stress from a spouse, particularly for the psychological symptoms and depression score. For those women assuming the caregiver role, the rates are all increased except in the presence of stress from children, which appears to have no marked additional impact. Multivariate analyses of these cross-sectional data consistently identified stress caused by a husband as a major factor for most of the health outcomes considered. Work appears to have a small health effect at best and has no role in explaining more acute health outcomes. The dominance of stress from a spouse as an additive effect, over and above the caregiver role, is a major finding, especially as the proportion of husbands causing stress is small.

SUMMARY AND DISCUSSION

Sparse evidence has been available regarding the beneficial nature of employment for women. It is remarkable that, in this randomly selected cohort of middle-aged women, from a general Massachusetts population, the evidence suggests a beneficial effect of continued employment that is unaffected by the menopausal transition and aging of the cohort by four years. Moreover, following the prior report from this same study by Jennings et al. (1984), the analyses reported and

Table 8.8 The Percentage Distribution of Three Acute Health Outcomes, by Presence of: Caregiver Role, Stress from Children and Stress from a Spouse

Caregiver	No				Yes			
Stress from children/husband	Neither	Children	Husband	Both	Neither	Children	Husband	Both
Health Outcomes								
1+ Physical symptoms	31.4	43.3	42.4	57.1	37.8	45.2	64.3	50.0
1+ Psychological symptoms	27.9	45.9	54.5	28.6	35.0	45.2	78.6	50.0
CES-D score ≥ 16	5.8	14.7	20.6	28.6	12.9	12.9	35.7	100.0
Total (100%)	925	194	66	7	323	62	14	2

summarized in this chapter do not merely support a healthy worker effect, but suggest that work may be beneficial in the face of stress from nurturing roles.

Those women in the employed/unemployed, intermittently employed, and continuously unemployed groups were similar in elevated reporting of symptoms, new chronic conditions, restricted activity days, and worse health. Despite these similarities and apparently worse perceived health at baseline, there was no consistent, significant deterioration in health for these groups. Moreover, there was no evidence that the burden of additional roles (and resulting stress) prevented women from participating in the labor force. Perhaps the most remarkable finding presented here is that women appear to work *despite* the presence of multiple nurturing roles that are frequent sources of stress.

These findings raise some interesting questions concerning how women manage multiple roles and the stresses that they may cause. At least for the variables considered, these factors have remarkably little impact on health. Work may play a protective role that is not entirely explained as a "healthy-worker" selection bias. Certainly, in any future research on the impact of employment on health—at least in middle-aged women—the presence of multiple family roles and the perceived function of work in relation to these roles must be considered. As expressed recently by Anesheusel (1986, p. 112): "It is not marriage per se or employment per se that impacts on a woman's psychological state, but the quality of her experience within these roles—the extent to which those roles provide her with a sense that she is valued and accepted by others, that she is satisfactorily meeting the expectations of others and that they are meeting her expectations." Work, with its clear expectations may provide a sense of satisfaction and self worth not equaled by the familial nurturing roles, for which expectations are implicit and more ambiguous.

Perhaps the most important findings regarding the impact of nurturing roles is the persistent effect of stress from a spouse. The literature is replete with reports of the positive effect of the presence of a wife on men's health. Almost no research has been reported on the impact of a husband on women's health. Separate analyses of the same data set indicate that approximately one-third of married women do not mention their husbands as members of their support network. It is a subset of these women who identify husbands as a source of stress.

Further research on the differing roles of a spouse for men and women is needed. Certainly the findings reported here indicate that the presence of a spouse may have very different effects on health for women, compared to men, especially in the presence of other nurturing roles. When viewed in the context of the two theoretical perspectives offered by Lewin-Epstein (1986), the results presented here also suggest perhaps a third more positive perspective on the work role. Rather than increasing role demand or constraining role obligations, work may actually alleviate the stress of nurturing roles and thus prevent morbidity.

REFERENCES

Anesheusel, C. (1986). Marital and employment role-strain, social support, and depression among adult women (pp. 99–114). In S. F. Hobfol (Ed.), *Stress, Social Support and Women*. New York: Hemisphere Publishing.

Brody, E. M. (1981). Women in the middle and family help to older people. *The Gerontologist, 25,* 19–29.

Cochrane, R., & Stope-Roe, M. (1981). Women, marriage, employment and mental health. *Br J Psychiatry, 139,* 373–381.

Croog, S., & Levine S. (1977). *The heart patient recovers*. New York: Behavioral Publications.

Gove, W., & Geerken, M. (1977). The effect of children and employment on the mental health of married men and women. *Social Forces, 56*(1), 67–77.

Gove, W., & Hughes, M. (1979). Possible causes of the apparent sex differences in physical health: An empirical investigation. *Am Soc Rev., 44,* 126.

Gove, W., & Tudor, J. (1973). Adult sex roles and mental illness. *Am J Sociol., 78,* 812.

Grossman A. S. (1977). The labor force patterns of divorcees and separated women. *Monthly Labor Review,* 48–53.

Haynes, S. G., Feinleib, M., & Levine, S. (1978). The relationship of psychosocial factors to coronary heart disease in the Framingham Study II. *Am J Epi., 107,* 384–402.

Haynes, S. G., & Feinleib, M. (1980). Women, work, and coronary heart disease: Prospective findings from the Framingham heart study. *Am J Pub Health, 70,* 133–141.

Hauensten, L. S., Kasl, S. V., & Harburg, E. (1977). Work status, work satisfaction, and blood pressure among married black and white women. *Psych of Women Quarterly, 1,* 334–349.

Howell, M. C. (1973). Employed mothers and their families. *Pediatrics, 52,* 252–263

Jaszmann, L. (1969). The perimenopausal symptoms. *Medical Gynecology and Sociology, 4,* 268–277.

Jennings, S., Mazaik, C., & McKinlay, S.(1984). Women and work: An investigation of the association between health and employment status in mid-aged women. *Soc Sci Med, 19*(4), 423–431.

Lewin-Epstein, N. (1986). Employment and ill-health in women in Israel. *Soc Sci Med, 23*(11), 1171–1179.

Maddox, G. L. (1964). Self-assessment of health status: a longitudinal study of selected elderly subjects. *J Chron Dis, 17,* 449–460.

Magursky, V., Mesko, M., & Sokolik, I. (1975). Age at menopause and onset of the climacteric in women of Martin District, Czechoslovakia. *Intn'l Journal of Fertility, 20,* 17–23.

Marcus, A. C., & Seeman, T. E. (1981). Sex differences in reports of illness and disability: a preliminary test of the fixed role obligations hypothesis. *Hlth Soc Behav, 22,* 124–82.

McKinlay, J. B., McKinlay, S. M., & Brambilla, D. J. (1987). Health status and utilization behavior associated with menopause. *Am J Epi.* 125, 110–121.

McKinlay, J., Tennstedt, S. (1986). Social Networks and the Care of Frail Elders, final report to the National Institute on Aging, grant no. AG03869, Boston, MA: Boston University.

McKinlay, S. M., Bifano, N. L., & McKinlay, J. B. (1985). Smoking and age at menopause. *Ann of Intern Med, 103,* 350–356.

Meisenhelder, J. B. (1986). Self-esteem in women: the influence of employment and perception of husband's appraisals. Image: *Journal of Nursing Scholarship, 18*(1), 8–14.

Mostow, E., & Newberry, P. (1975). Work role and depression in women: a comparison of workers and housewives in treatment. *Am J Orthopsychiatry, 45,* 538–544.

Nathanson, C. A. (1975). Illness and the feminine role: a theoretical view. *Soc Soci Med, 9,* 57–62.

Nathanson, C. A. (1980). Social roles and health status among women: the significance on employment. *Soc Sci Med, 14,* 463.

Parry, G. (1986). Paid employment, life events, social support, and mental health in working class mothers. *J Health Soc Behav, 27*(2), 193–208.

Radloff, L. S. (1977). The CES-D Scale: A self-report depression scale for research in the general population. *App Psych Measurement, 1,* 385–401.

Rice, D. P., & Cugliani, A. S. (1979). Health status of American women (pp. 72–78) in Proceedings of the American Statistical Association (Social Statistics Section). Washington, DC: American Statistical Association.

Treloar, A. E. (1974). Menarche, menopause, and intervening fecundability. *Human Biology, 46,* 89–107.

U.S. Department of Labor. (1985). Office of the Secretary, Women's Bureau: United Nations Decade for Women, 1976–1985: Employment in the United States. Washington, DC: U.S. Government Printing Office.

Verbrugge, L. (1985). Gender and health: An update on hypotheses and evidence. *J Hlth and Soc Beh, 26,* 156–182.

Verbrugge, L. (1983). Multiple roles and physical health of women and men. *J of Health, 24,* 16–30.

Waldron, I. (1978). The coronary-prone behavior pattern, blood pressure, employment, and socio-economic status in women. *J of Psychosomatic Research, 22,* 79–87.

Waldron, I., Herold, J., Donn, D., & Staum, R. (1982). Reciprocal effects of health and labor force participation among women: evidence from two longitudinal studies. *J Occ Med, 24*(2), 126–132.

Welch, S., & Booth, A. (1977). Employment and health among married women. *Sex Roles, 3,* 385.

Woods, N. F., & Hulka, B. S. (1979). Symptom reports and illness behavior among employed women and homemakers. *J Comm Health, 5,* 36.

9 Gender and the Use of Health Services among Elderly Persons

Cynthia Thomas
Howard R. Kelman

Men and women have different health problems. Men have higher rates of serious, potentially fatal diseases; women, higher rates of generally nonfatal illnesses and chronic conditions. Whether these differences are due primarily to biology or to psychosocial factors influenced by their different gender roles in life is unclear but widely debated. Similarly, rates of health service use have been found to differ between men and women. Men tend to be hospitalized more often (Mutran & Ferraro, 1988; Roos & Shapiro, 1981; Verbrugge & Wingard, 1986; Waddell & Floate, 1986; Wolinsky, Mosely, & Coe, 1986), perhaps at least in part because their illnesses, especially those related to heart disease, often are more serious. Women, however, visit physicians more frequently (Homan & Haddock, 1986; Kronenfeld, 1980; Mossey, 1985; Mutran & Ferraro, 1988; Verbrugge & Vingard, 1986), perhaps because they practice more preventive care, or because they more often have chronic conditions that require monitoring.

Many studies on health and health service use of men and women have focused on adults of all ages, or have combined those 65 years and older into a single-age category. Often, only a few key services have been examined, even though there may be other services frequently used by either men or women. This chapter examines differences in patterns of health service use among men and women aged 65 to 98, across a full range of services, using data from a longitudinal study of health and aging conducted in Bronx, New York.

This work supported by a grant from the National Institute on Aging, P01 AG03424.

DIFFERENCES IN HEALTH AND HEALTH SERVICE USE

Although rates of a few conditions, such as migraine headaches, decrease with age for both sexes, most conditions are present at higher rates as people age, such that the elderly are disproportionately represented in hospital beds. Some health changes appear to bring men and women closer together as they pass age 65, such as higher rates of coronary heart disease, hypertension, and visual and hearing impairments among women, and, among men, higher rates of constipation, gall bladder, thyroid conditions, and urinary tract disorders (Verbrugge, 1985). In general, however, women remain sicker (Wingard, 1984; Verbrugge, Chapter 10, this volume). Of course, most data on disease conditions by gender and age are based on cross-sectional data, which means that comparisons between people aged 45 to 65 and 65 and over, for example, are confounded by cohort effects. Hence, one sees that rates of emphysema are considerably higher for women 45 to 65 than for women over 65, because the younger women are more often smokers and presumably will carry their higher rates of emphysema along with them as they age.

Women also seem to experience certain mental symptoms more than men, especially depression; whether this is due to genetic or psychosocial factors, or both, is unknown (Dohrenwend & Dohrenwend, 1976). At all ages, women are more often under treatment for depression but are also more likely to report feeling depressed in community-based studies (Weissman & Klerman, 1981). In younger women, depression is sometimes related to the reproductive process, especially the postpartum period; there is mixed opinion about the impact of menopause (Weissman & Klerman, 1981). Using the Center for Epidemiologic Studies Depression Scale (CES-D) as a measure, there is some indication that both sexes have the same underlying types of symptoms of depression, but with different rank orders of importance (Clark, Aneshensel, Frerichs, & Morgan, 1981). On the other hand, differences in specific symptoms of depression may be important across age groups, rather than by gender (Clark et al., 1981).

Although reasons for differences in health between older men and women are not well understood, other characteristics of men and women appear to converge with age, including some of the role differences that are thought to affect health service use. Injuries, more common among younger men than women, occur at more equal rates at older ages, as exposure to risky activities declines for men, and women begin to suffer the falls and hip fractures associated with osteoporosis. After a certain age, women no longer visit doctors and hospitals because of pregnancy. Both men and women are likely to be at home rather than working, and to share, more nearly, the same concerns about daily living. They also have an equivalent amount of time available for medical visits. Considering these factors the net effect on health service use might be an elimination of gender differences, if psychosocial factors predominate, or an increase in gender differences if health factors predominate.

Because people over 65 and, indeed, those over 85 are among the most rapidly increasing segments of the population today, it is important to obtain a better understanding of their use of health services. At every age level, women outnumber men. Over age 65, however, the rate at which women outnumber men accelerates until, at ages 75 to 79, there are more than 10 women for every 7 men and, over age 80, there are 10 women for every 5 men (US Bureau of Census, 1986). Consequently, it is important not only to understand health service use among the elderly at various age levels, but also to compare service use between men and women. Perhaps we can learn from any unequal service use between the sexes how to provide more efficient health service for everyone in order to decrease rates of illness and disability and improve longevity.

STUDY SAMPLE

Data presented here are taken from interviews conducted as part of the Norwood Aging Study (NAS). The study consisted of 1855 men and women at minimum 65 years old who were randomly selected from a list of Medicare beneficiaries living in a defined geographic area, one mile in diameter, in the north central section of the Bronx. This area was chosen for its relatively high proportion of elderly residents in 1980 (20%), and because of the availability to residents of several well-established health service delivery systems and hospitals. The interviews took place between July 1984 and March 1985, and are the first in a series of semiannual interviews conducted as part of a longitudinal aging study (Kelman & Thomas, 1988).

Men and women in this sample were born between 1886 and 1919; 10.8% were born in the 19th century. Approximately 40% were born outside the United States, especially in western Europe, with a large percentage coming from Ireland. The men and women differ, however, in important respects according to other characteristics. The mean number of years of employment is 44.9 for men and 24.2 for women. Fourteen percent of the men and 8% of the women are still working today, although they have passed the customary retirement age of 65. Men in the sample were employed most often in technical and supervisory positions and women in clerical jobs. Over half the men are married today, but only 30% of the women have spouses. Almost twice as many women as men live alone.

Differences in economic resources are considerable. Approximately one-fourth of the women, but only 9% of men live on less than $5,000 a year. Sixteen percent of the women and 12% of the men receive Federal payments for medical care under Medicaid for expenses not covered by the Medicare program. These data are presented in Table 9.1.

HEALTH DIFFERENCES BETWEEN MEN AND WOMEN

The rates of 13 chronic conditions, generally most common or troublesome among elderly people, are reported in Table 9.2 in columns labeled NAS. Comparable data from the 1984 Health Interview Survey's Supplement on Aging are shown in columns labeled SOA. Women in the study sample more often report having been told by a doctor that they have four of the conditions—arthritis or rheumatism, hypertension, varicose veins, and a broken hip. Men in the study sample lead in only two, but both of them are extremely serious: heart attacks and coronary heart disease.

The national data also show similar total rates and higher rates for women for arthritis or rheumatism, hypertension, and broken hips, three of the four conditions. The sample from the Bronx, however, reports varicose veins approximately twice as often as the national sample, although differences between men and women are comparable. Other than varicose veins, the frequency of various reported conditions among men and women are close to national estimates in the Bronx sample.

Sixteen percent of the men in the Bronx sample, but only 9% of the women, reported the absence of any physical conditions, as shown in Table 9.3. A few more women than men had five conditions or more. Symptoms of two types of mental problems were measured— depression and cognitive impairment. Higher proportions of women than men responded affirmatively to questions indicating depressive symptomatology; the number of men and women showing signs of possible cognitive impairment are similar.

Respondents were asked to report on their difficulties, if any, in performing nine daily activities: going in or out of their houses or apartments; getting around inside their homes; climbing stairs; grasping faucets, door knobs, or pots on the stove; using bathroom facilities and kitchen equipment; getting in or out of bed; dressing; using a step stool; or using the telephone. Seventy-nine percent of the men, but only

Table 9.1 Characteristics of Men and Women in the Sample[a]

Characteristic	Men	Women
Mean age (years)	75.0	75.5
65–74	49.5	48.4
75–84	40.2	40.8
85+	10.4	10.9
Ethnicity: nonwhite,	4.8	5.3
Hispanic	5.4	5.7
Currently married	60.3*	30.7
One person household	26.8	51.0*
Education (9+ years)	61.1	57.8
Median income ($)	11,500	7,400
Mean income ($)	15,257*	10,276
<5,000	9.2	23.1*
5–15,000	57.8	59.3
>15,000	33.0*	17.6
Medicaid	11.5	16.2*
Medicare Part B[b]	95.2*	91.9
Private health insurance	71.8*	66.2
Employment		
Currently working full or part time	14.3*	8.2
Mean years worked	44.9*	24.2
Worked at least one year	96.4*	81.5
Occupation		
Supervisory, technical	30.0	15.1
Craftsperson	17.2	3.5
Service workers	11.9	20.3
Clerical	13.4	34.7
Other	27.5	26.4
Self-Assessed Health: Fair/Poor	37.5	43.4*
Birthplace		
United States	59.6	56.9
Bronx	10.8	9.3
Elsewhere	48.8	47.6
Outside United States	40.4	43.1
West Europe, Canada	20.3	21.3
East Europe	17.0	18.6
Central, South America, Carribean	2.2	2.5
Asia	0.9	0.7
Total	584	1271
Percentage	31.5	68.5

[a]Percentages, means and all other calculations in this and subsequent tables are based on weighted data; totals are unweighted. Weights were applied for unequal probability sampling. Values represent percentages unless otherwise noted.
[b]Optional coverage for physician services.
*Gender difference is significant at $p < .05$ by t-test.

Table 9.2 Selected Medical Conditions: Study sample (NAS)[1] and Health Interview Survey Supplement on Aging (SOA)[2] (percentages)

Characteristic	Age (Years)															
	65-74				75-84				85 & Over				Total			
	SOA		NAS		SOA		NAS		SOA		NAS		SOA		NAS	
	M	W	M	W	M	W	M	W	M	W	M	W	M	W	M	W
Diseases Reported																
Arthritis and rheumatism	43.2	55.6	36.8	56.8	42.9	60.9	36.7	58.8	39.1	57.9	44.4	62.7	42.9	57.6	37.5	58.2
Hypertension	37.9	46.0	36.6	47.0	34.2	53.0	36.0	49.8	32.1	48.7	32.5	40.8	36.5	48.5	35.9	47.5
Varicose veins	6.5	12.8	14.0	20.6	4.7	12.2	12.4	22.0	5.5	11.8	13.4	17.5	5.9	12.5	13.3	20.8
Arteriosclerosis	10.0	7.9	10.4	8.1	12.3	13.7	13.0	15.1	19.1	23.4	14.5	20.1	11.2	11.1	11.9	12.2
Diabetes	10.5	10.2	10.9	10.6	10.0	10.0	12.1	13.7	5.5	6.8	12.1	7.6	10.1	9.9	11.5	11.6
Heart attack	11.0	5.7	14.2	8.7	10.5	7.7	13.4	9.8	6.6	9.7	13.3	10.6	10.6	6.7	13.8	9.4
Angina	6.9	6.7	8.4	9.5	7.5	7.0	10.9	10.8	4.0	7.1	7.2	13.5	6.9	6.8	9.3	10.5
Cancer	11.0	10.9	8.4	12.0	14.7	11.9	11.5	10.3	14.3	12.3	6.0	8.8	12.2	11.3	9.4	11.0
Broken hip	1.4	2.8	3.6	3.4	2.9	6.1	3.1	5.9	6.8	11.2	7.3	12.4	2.1	4.6	3.8	5.4
Osteoporosis	0.7	4.9	2.3	6.7	0.4	5.5	3.4	9.3	1.2	5.8	3.7	5.8	0.6	5.2	2.9	7.7
Stroke	6.4	4.1	5.6	4.7	9.0	7.8	5.6	4.7	7.8	12.1	7.2	5.3	7.2	6.0	5.8	4.8
Coronary disease	7.1	2.7	6.7	2.9	6.2	3.6	3.7	3.6	6.1	4.2	9.6	6.4	6.8	3.1	5.8	3.6
Altzheimer's disease	*	*	*	*	*	*	*	*	*	*	*	*	*	*	*	*

*< .5% for SOA data; < 2.6% for NAS data.

[1]NAS question: "Has a doctor ever told . . .?"; SOA question: "Have you ever had . . .?"

[2]Data are weighted up to United States estimates and are based on runs prepared by Dr. Jack Guralnik, Epidemiology, Demography and Biometry Program, NIA.

Table 9.3 Functional Status by Age and Gender (Percentages)

	Age (Years)							
Characteristic	65–74		75–84		85 & Over		Total	
	M	W	M	W	M	W	M	W
Number of reported medical conditions								
0	16.8	10.8	16.2	8.1	15.7	8.2	16.4	9.4
5+	8.1	6.7	5.9	13.4	8.4	9.9	7.3	10.0
Sensory difficulties								
Vision—some/a lot	26.3	30.4	37.3	46.0	50.6	58.2	33.3	40.0
Hearing—some/a lot	29.8	23.8	39.8	35.7	56.6	52.1	36.6	31.7
Symptoms of depression (CES-D)[a]	9.6	16.5	13.3	21.5	10.6	30.7	11.2	19.9
Symptoms of congitive impairment (MMSE)[b]	12.2	13.3	22.3	30.8	54.4	52.6	20.5	24.4
Number of activities that are difficult								
0	83.6	76.7	79.1	66.7	55.6	39.3	79.0	68.7
3+	5.5	8.3	7.5	15.8	19.8	42.9	7.8	15.0
Number of activities requiring help								
0	94.0	87.3	88.1	78.8	74.1	53.0	89.6	80.2
3+	4.3	4.9	2.2	7.8	8.6	28.0	3.9	8.6
Any days in bed in past 2 weeks	7.3	12.0	6.9	8.7	7.3	14.6	7.1	10.9
Self-assessed health:								
fair or poor	34.2	40.5	38.7	46.3	51.3	45.3	37.7	43.4
worse now than a year ago	18.5	23.1	22.9	27.7	31.2	38.0	21.5	26.5
Control over health								
Little or None	24.5	24.8	24.6	29.9	40.8	41.7	26.1	28.6

[a]Score of 16 or higher on Center for Epidemiologic Studies Depression Scale (CES-D).
[b]Score below 18 on Mini-Mental State Examination (MMSE).

69% of the women, reported no difficulty with any activity. A similar series of seven questions on functional limitations from the 1984 National Health Interview Survey yielded 81.3% of males age 65 and over and 74.6% of females with no reported difficulties in daily activities (NCHS, 1987).

Approximately 14% of the women and 8% of the men had difficulty with three or more of the items. Most of these health and functional differences are present for men and women in each of three age categories: 65 to 74, 75 to 84, and 85 and over. Summary measures, then, indicate that women in the samples are less healthy than men, in terms of their ability to function satisfactorily in daily living and the number of medical conditions they report. This is similar to comparable national data.

Health problems have been found to be the most significant predictors of health care utilization (Branch et al., 1981; Ory & Bond, 1989; Soldo & Manton, 1985; Wan, 1982; Wolinsky, 1984), and on the basis of health alone one might expect that women in this sample would use more health services than men. Other factors shown to be associated with the use of health services include the level of available economic resources, age, whether one lives alone or with others, and ethnicity, with blacks typically using fewer resources than whites (Soldo & Manton, 1985; Wan, 1982; Wolinsky, 1984). For all of these characteristics, except age and ethnicity, women in the sample have traits disposing them either to overutilize or to underutilize health services in relation to men. Women more often live alone, which may lead to greater use of services. Their lower incomes and rates of private insurance coverage should tend to discourage use; on the other hand, higher proportions of women than men receive Medicaid, which covers virtually all charges for medical care and is likely to encourage service use. Roughly equivalent age and ethnicity distributions should not affect rates of service use by men and women differentially, although age and ethnicity may interact with gender to produce different effects on service use for one sex or the other. It is not clear what the net impact of all of these characteristics on service use is likely to be. If these contradictory differences between men and women in health and psychosocial factors are taken into account, will differences in health services utilization disappear?

HEALTH SERVICE USE

Unlike many studies of health service use among men and women, this one examines a full range of services. Three major categories of health service were considered: hospitalizations, ambulatory care visits, and use of health-related services. Ambulatory care includes not only physician visits, but visits to emergency rooms, outpaient clinics, and all other health care visits, including any visits for tests, shots, or other procedures. Intensity of hospital use was measured by total days of hospitalization and average length of stay. The health-related services are meals-on-wheels, senior center meals, special transportation for the elderly, homemaker services, telephone monitoring, shopping, visiting nurses, home health aides, and money management.

There were six categories of independent or predictor variables: (1) health (including number of conditions, number of problems of daily living, whether self-perceived health was either good to excellent, or fair to poor, and whether self-perceived health was worse today than a year ago); (2) mental health status (symptoms of depression and cognitive impairment); (3) age; (4) levels of available economic resources (per capita income, Medicaid status, and coverage by private insurance); (5) ethnicity (nonwhite or not, Hispanic or not); and (6) living arrangements (whether living alone or with others).

First, we examined whether men and women differed in their rates of use of each service or intensity of hospital use, comparing unadjusted mean use rates. Men have significantly higher mean rates of hospitalization overall, and among those hospitalized at least once, men also have higher mean hospitalization rates than comparable women (as shown in Table 9.4). Once hospitalized, however, men and women remain for equivalent numbers of mean and total days.

Women, on average, use more health-related services and are more likely than men to have visited a physician at least once in a 3 month period. Rates of other visits for ambulatory care—to emergency rooms, outpatient clinics, or to any other places—are no different for men and women when means are compared, so that women's higher rate of use of ambulatory care, overall, is accounted for primarily by physician visits. Table 9.4 also indicates the amount of overlap in the distributions of use rates (standard deviations). Where there is greater overlap in distributions of rates of use across genders, there may also be a greater likelihood that factors other than gender account for at least some of the differences. These straightforward comparisons of means, then, do not necessarily reveal important differences in patterns of health-service use between men and women.

As a first step in examining whether these mean differences are actually due to other characteristics of men and women that differ, the independent variable, gender, was regressed on each of the dependent utilization variables. We used a series of ordinary least squares regression equations, taking the logarithm of the dependent utilization variables (numbers of visits), which are skewed to the right, to make the distributions conform to the assumptions of the model. The results, shown in Table 9.5, column 1, confirm the findings concerning differences in mean utilization rates shown in Table 9.4. Men and women differ in their rates of use of three specific medical services: hospitals (in-patient), private physicians, and health-related services. The duration of hospital stays and other types of ambulatory care use rates are essentially equivalent across gender. Women, however, make more visits than men when all types of ambulatory care are summed together.

We next examined whether these male–female differences in utiliza-

Table 9.4 Gender Differences in Utilization of Health Services

Measures of health service use	Men X̄	Men SD	Women X̄	Women SD	Total X̄	Total SD
Hospital inpatient (past 12 Months)						
Rate of Hospitalization	0.4[+]	1.3	0.3	0.7	0.3	0.9
Hospitalized—one or more times (%)	22.0*	10.0	18.8	13.9	19.5	17.1
Mean no. of hospitalizations per person hospitalized	1.7[+]	2.3	1.4	0.8	1.5	1.6
Mean no. of days per person hospitalized	23.9	34.1	22.6	29.2	23.1	31.1
Mean length of stay per hospitalization	13.7	28.4	16.0	26.7	15.0	27.4
Ambulatory care (Past 3 Months)						
Total ambulatory care visits[a]						
One or more visits (%)	56.0	12.0	65.9*	16.9	62.6	20.8
Mean no. of visits for ambulatory care of those who made ambulatory care visits	4.5	9.2	3.8	7.3	4.0	7.9
Emergency room visits						
One or more visits (%)	10.0	7.2	9.6	10.5	9.7	12.7
Mean no. of visits of those who used emergency rooms	1.5	1.7	1.3	0.8	1.4	1..2
Outpatient clinics						
One or more visits (%)	15.1	8.6	14.5	12.6	14.7	15.3
Mean no. of visits of those who used O.P.D.'s	3.3	6.0	2.8	4.5	3.0	5.1
Private physician visits						
One or more visits (%)	38.5	1.8	50.9*	17.8	46.7	21.5
Mean no. of visits of those who used private physicians	2.5	3.4	2.1	2.4	2.2	2.7
Other health care visits[b]						
One or more visits (%)	19.3	9.5	21.6	14.7	20.8	17.5
Mean no. of visits of those who used other providers	4.8	11.8	4.6	10.3	4.7	10.8
Health related services (past 12 Months)						
Rate of health-related services utilized	0.3	0.8	0.5[+]	1.0	0.4	1.0
One or more services (%)	17.9	9.3	26.4*	15.7	23.6	18.3
Mean no. of services of those who used health-related services	1.7	1.1	1.9	1.2	1.8	1.2
Total	584		1271		1855	
Percentage	33.7		66.3		100	

[a]The sum of all visits to emergency rooms, outpatient clinics, private physicians and other health care providers.
[b]Includes visits to psychiatrists, other mental health professionals, other therapists and visits for diagnostic testing.
*Gender difference is significant at $p < .05$ by Chi-square analysis.
[+]Gender difference is significant at $p < .05$ by t-test.

tion rates—hospitalizations, physician visits, health related service use, and total ambulatory care—would remain when controlling for each of the six categories of predictor variables alone, again using multiple regression analysis. Specifically, we asked whether the effect of gender on utilization would disappear in the presence of any one particular type of predictor variable; that is, whether either physical health, mental health status, age, level of economic resources, living alone or not or, finally, ethnicity, could be said to account for the gender differences. (These results are reported in Table 9.5, columns 2 through 7.)

Health status, generally the most important reason for seeking out any form of medical care or service, does not cancel out the independent effects of gender on utilization for any single category of service usage, nor does any other type of predictor variable. That is, even accounting for differences in characteristics, men are hospitalized more often, women visit physicians more frequently, and use more health-related services.

However, poor physical and mental health appear to account for the greater frequency of the *total* number of ambulatory care visits by women. No other category of variables other than health cancels out women's higher visit rate. That is, the larger number of ambulatory visits by women is only accounted for by women's poorer health and not because women are older, poorer, or more often live alone than men. The implication of these findings is that gender plays a role in determining the specific type of ambulatory visit, but not the total number of such visits. The total number of visits is affected by both physical and mental health, but health plays no role in determining the place to visit.

We have seen that, although there are differences in use rates between men and women in three categories of service—hospitalizations, physician visits, and health-related service use—when controlling for a single set of variables at a time, there are no male–female differences in five other measures of use; mean length of hospital stay, total days in the hospital, number of emergency room visits, number of outpatient clinic visits (generally) and number of other health care visits. Also, we noted that differences between men and women in rates of total ambulatory care disappear when health variables are controlled. Although no single characteristic, such as poorer overall health of women or higher income among men eliminates the effect of gender on the three specific forms of service use, it is possible that the independent variables, in combination, might eliminate gender effects. In fact, we find that in only one of these three types of health care visits are we able to eliminate differences between men

Table 9.5 Gender Differences in Health Services Utilization: Gender Alone and with Each Control Variable Set[a,b]

Measures of health service use	Gender only	Gender and control variables					
		Mental health	Physical health	Age	Economic resources	Living arrangements	Ethnicity
Column:	1	2	3	4	5	6	7
Number of Hospitalizations	M*	M*	M*	M*	M*	M*	M*
Mean length of stay per person hospitalized	*	*	*	*	*	*	*
Total days in hospital for those hospitalized	*	*	*	*	*	*	*
Number of ambulatory care visits	F*	*	*	F*	F*	F*	F*
Number of emergency room visits	*	*	*	*	*	*	*
Number of outpatient clinic visits	*	M*	*	*	*	*	*
Number of private physician visits	F*	F*	F*	F*	F*	F*	F*
Number of other health care visits[c]	*	*	*	*	*	*	*
Number of health-related services utilized	F*	F*	F*	F*	F*	F*	F*

[a] In this and subsequent tables, the dependent variable in all regressions has been transformed by taking the logarithm of the original dependent variable.

[b] Variable Description:

Gender 1 if male, 0 otherwise

Mental Health Symptoms of depression: 0 if score on CES-D scale is under 16, 1 otherwise. Symptoms of mental impairment: 1 if score is under 18 on MMSE, 0 otherwise

Physical Health Number of conditions: continuous variable with a range of 0–17 Number of problems of daily living: continuous variable with a range of 0–9. Self-perceived health: 0 if good to excellent, 1 if fair or poor: 0 if the same or better than a year ago, 1 if worse.

Age Continuous variable, range: 65–98

Economic resources Per capita income with a range of $250–120,000. Medicaid status: 1 if enrolled, 0 otherwise, Private insurance: 1 if covered, 0 otherwise.

Ethnicity 1 if Black, 0 otherwise, 1 if Hispanic, 0 otherwise.

Living arrangements 1 if living alone, 0 otherwise.

[c] Includes visits to psychiatrists, other mental health professionals, other therapists and visits for diagnostic testing.

M = Utilization rate is higher for males than for females and gender/utilization relationship is significant at $p < .05$ by t-test.

F = Utilization rate is higher for females than for males and gender/utilization relationship is significant at $p < .05$ by t-test.

*Gender differences in utilization rates are not significant at $p < .05$ by t-test.

and women by controlling for more than one of the predictor variable sets simultaneously.

Table 9.6 shows the p value for gender as each new type of independent variable is added in step-wise regression equations for each of the three forms of health-service use. Even when all six categories of independent variables are included simultaneously in the equations, gender continues to remain significant for two of these three forms of utilization—men continue to show more hospitalizations, and women still visit doctors more often (see Table 9.6), as has been found in studies of men and women across the entire adult age range.

After controlling for the various other factors associated with service use, we see that women no longer receive more health-related services. We attempted to identify the most concise set of reasons for the disappearance of gender as a predictor of health-related service use. First, we ranked each set of variables according to the size of their coefficient of multiple correlation with health-service use, and then incorporated them a set at a time in a step-wise regression equation in order of the size of the coefficient. Health, economic resources, and age (variables with the three largest correlation coefficients) did not eliminate the effect of gender, but mental health, added to the other three, gave females and males equivalent rates of service use. A combination, then, of poorer health, fewer economic resources, age, and possible mental problems are the factors that contribute to greater utilization of health-related services by women.

Are we to conclude, then, that men, because they are men, are hospitalized more often than women, and that women, because they are women, visit doctors more often? We cannot be certain, of course, that we have measured all of the important aspects of health. We only measured two types of symptoms of mental disorder. The type and severity of medical conditions may not be fully captured in the summary health measures used here, and may affect hospitalizations and physician use. But severity variables and a complete set of mental health indicators have rarely been measured in other similar studies and their effect, if any, on utilization rates remains to be explored.

For each of the nine utilization variables, we ran separate regression equations for males and females to see whether the same factors (or different ones) were associated with increasing levels of service use. We examined each specific independent variable within the categories of health, mental health status, level of economic resources, and ethnicity, as well as age and whether living alone or with others. Results are presented in Table 9.7.

Considering, first, the two categories of service use in which we found greater use by either males or females—numbers of hospitaliza-

Table 9.6 Gender Differences in Health Services Utilization: Results of Step-wise Regression Analyses

Hospitalizations		Private Physician Visits		Health-related Services	
Use Rate: M > W	*p* Value: Gender	Use Rate: W > M	*p* Value: Gender	Use Rate: M = W	*p* Value: Gender
Health	.001	Health	.02	Health	.009
+ Mental Health	.001	+ Mental Health	.05	+ Economic Resources	.05
+ Age	.001	+ Economic Resources	.02	+ Age	.04
+ Economic Resources	.001	+ Ethnicity	.02	+ Mental Health	.12
+ 2+ household size	.001	+ Age	.02	+ 2+ household size	.87
+ Ethnicity	.001	+ 2+ household size	.01	+ Ethnicity	.88
$R^2 = .10$		$R^2 = .11$		$R^2 = .27$	

Table 9.7 Gender Differences in Factors Affecting Utilization

Measures of health service use	Men		Women	
	R^2	Characteristics	R^2	Characteristics[a]
Rate of hospitalization	.14	Nonwhite Number of conditions Self-assessed health worse than 1 year ago Problems of daily living (PDL)	.08	Number of conditions self-assessed health worse than 1 year ago Problems of daily living (PDL)
Total days in hospital for those hospitalized	.26	Self-assessed Health: fair/poor Problems of daily living (PDL) Medicaid	.08	Hispanic
Mean length of stay per person hospitalized	.25	Nonwhite (−) Problems of daily living (PDL)	.09	Hispanic (−) Per capita income[b]
Rate of ambulatory care visits	.18	Number of conditions Problems of daily living (PDL) Symptoms of depression (CES-D) Medicaid Supplemental insurance	.16	Number of conditions Problems of daily living (PDL) Symptoms of depression (CES-D) Medicaid Age (−) Self-assessed health worse than 1 year ago
Rate of emergency room visits	.09	Problems of daily living (PDL) Symptoms of depression (CES-D) Self-assessed health worse than 1 year ago Hispanic	.05	Problems of daily living (PDL) Symptoms of depression (CES-D) CES-D Score missing[c] Number of conditions
Rate of outpatient clinic visits	.09	Number of conditions Nonwhite Symptoms of depression (CES-D) Medicaid	.08	Number of conditions Nonwhite Self-assessed health worse than 1 year ago

Health service	R^2	Predictors (column 1)	R^2	Predictors (column 2)	Predictors (column 3)
Rate of private physician visits	.10	Number of conditions; CES-D score missing; Supplemental insurance	.12	Number of conditions; CES-D score missing (−); Supplemental insurance; Medicaid; Symptoms of depression (CES-D)	CES-D score missing; Supplemental insurance; Age (−); Hispanic
Rate of other health care visits[d]	.16	Number of conditions; Problems of daily living (PDL); Symptoms of depression (CES-D); Symptoms of congitive impairment (MMSE) (−)	.08	Number of conditions; Problems of daily living (PDL); Symptoms of depression (CES-D)	Age (−); 2+ household size; Self-assessed health: Fair/Poor
Rate of health-related services utilized	.22	Problems of daily living (PDL); Medicaid; Age; 2+ household size (−); Symptoms of depression (CES-D)	.29	Problems of daily living (PDL); Medicaid; Age; 2+ household size (−)	Per Capita Income; Hispanic; Number of conditions; Self-assessed health: Fair/Poor; Self-assessed health worse than 1 year ago

[a] Significantly related to health-service use at $p < .05$ by t-test. Relationship is positive unless followed by (−).
[b] Per capita income for spousal household obtained by dividing total income for both spouses in half.
[c] Incomplete or no CES-D data obtained.
[d] Includes visits to psychiatrists, other mental health professionals, other therapists, and visits for diagnostic testing.

tions and visits to physicians—we find, in each case, that similar factors affect utilization. The health variables—in particular, number of conditions, whether one's health is worse on the day of the interview than it was a year earlier, and the number of functional limitations—were related to the number of hospitalizations for both sexes. In general, many of the same types of variables appear to explain ambulatory care use for both men and women, particularly health measures, although different individual variables are important for different utilization measures for men and women. Number of conditions is important in every category of service use for women, and in all categories of service use except visits to the emergency room and number of health-related services for men. Mental health problems—in particular, an unfavorable score on a screen for depression—is related to total ambulatory care, emergency room visits and "other" visits (which include mental health visits) for both men and women. For all utilization measures except those related to hospital visits, many of the same variables explain use for both men and women, but several additional variables are significant for women. Age, for example, is negatively associated with use of outpatient clinic visits, other health care visits, and total ambulatory care for women but not for men, suggesting that older women may find it difficult or unnecessary to obtain certain forms of care, in contrast to men or younger women.

SUMMARY AND CONCLUSIONS

Initially, we found differences in four types of health service use between men and women over age 65: in rates of hospitalizations, physician visits, health-related service use, and in rates of total ambulatory care. We found, however, that women make more ambulatory visits, altogether, than men, only because they are sicker. Even accounting for differences in health and psychosocial factors, men still are hospitalized more often than women, and women are found to visit physicians more frequently than men. Differences in health-related service use are accounted for by a combination of four factors: physical health, availability of economic resources, age, and mental health (depression).

By implication, women's greater use of physicians' services often has been defined as overuse, whereas men's more frequent hospitalizations are attributed to the severity of their illnesses. Explanations such as availability of more leisure time and greater sensitivity to symptoms often read as thinly veiled substitutes for the word hypochondriasis for women; men are not similarly accused of malingering. Indeed, findings presented here suggest many similarities in health service use between men and women, especially with respect to the factors associated with total numbers of visits for ambulatory care, which for both, are primarily physical health, symptoms of depression, and availability of economic resources. Although older men and women may use individual types of health services at different rates, at equivalent levels of health, both use equivalent amounts of ambulatory care overall.

REFERENCES

Branch, L. A., Jette, A. M., Evaschwick, M., Polansky, M., Rowe, G., & Diehr, P. (1981). Toward understanding elders' health services utilization. *Journal of Community Health, 7,* 80.

Clark, V. A., Aneshensel, C. S., Frerichs, R. R., & Morgan, T. M. (1981). Analysis of effects of sex and age in response to items on the CES-D scale. *Psychiatry Research, 5,* 171.

Dohrenwend, B. P., & Dohrenwend, B. S. (1976). Sex differences and psychiatric disorders. *American Journal of Sociology, 81*(6), 1447.

Homan, S., & Haddock, C. (1986). Widowhood, sex, labor force participation and use of physician services by elderly adults. *Journal of Gerontology, 27,* 332.

Kelman, H. R., & Thomas, C. T. (1988). Hospital and ambulatory service use by the urban elderly under different health care delivery systems. *Medical Care, 26*(8), 739–749.

Kronenfeld, J. J. (1980). Sources of ambulatory care and utilization models. *Health Services Research, 15,* 3.

Mossey, J. M. (1985). Physician use by the elderly over an eight-year period. *American Journal of Public Health, 75,* 1333.

Mutran, E., & Ferraro, K. F. (1988). Medical need and the use of services among older men and women. *Journal of Gerontology, 48*(5), S162.

National Center for Health Statistics, Dawson, B., Hendershot, G., & Fulton, J. (1987). Aging in the eighties, functional limitations of individuals age 65 years and over. *Advance Data from Vital Health Statistics* (p. 3). No. 133. DHHS Pub. No. (PHS) 87-1250. Public Health Service. Hyattsville, MD: U.S. Government Printing Office.

Ory, M., & Bond, K. (Eds.). (1989). *Aging and health care: Social science and policy perspectives.* New York: Routledge.

Roos, N. P., & Shapiro, E. (1981). The Manitoba longitudinal study on aging. *Medical Care, 19,* 651.

Soldo, B. J., & Manton, K. G. (1985). Health status and service needs of the oldest old: Current patterns and future trends. *Health and Society, 63,* 286.

United States Bureau of the Census. (1986). *Statistical abstract of the United States: 1987* (107th ed., p. 18). Washington, DC: U.S. Government Printing Office.

Verbrugge, L. (1985). Gender and health: An update on hypotheses and evidence. *Journal of Health and Social Behavior, 26,* 159.

Verbrugge, L. (1990). The Twain meet: Empirical explanations of sex differences in health and mortality. In M. G. Ory & H. R. Warner (Eds.), *Gender, health, and longevity: Multidisciplinary perspectives* (pp. 159–199). New York: Springer Publishing Co.

Verbrugge, L. M., & Wingard, D. L. (1986). Sex differentials in health and mortality. In A. H. Stromberg (Ed.), *Women, health, and medicine* (pp. 60–82). Palo Alto, CA: Mayfield Publishing Co.

Waddell, C., & Floate, P. (1986). Research note: Gender and utilization of health care services in Perth, Australia. *Sociology, Health, and Illness, 8,* 170.

Wan, T. T. H. (1982). Use of health services by the elderly in low-income communities. *Milbank Memorial Fund Quarterly, 60,* 82.

Weissman, M. M., & Klerman, G. L. (1981). Sex differences and the epidemiology of depression. In E. Howell, & M. Bayes (Eds.), *Women and mental health* (p. 160). New York: Basic Books.

Wingard, D. L. (1984). The sex differential in morbidity, mortality, and life style. *American Review of Public Health, 5,* 433–458.

Wolinsky, F. D. (1984). Physician and hospital utilization among noninstitutionalized elderly adults: An analysis of the health interview survey. *Journal of Gerontology, 89,* 334.

Wolinsky, F. D., Mosely, R., & Coe, R. (1986). A cohort analysis of the use of health services by elderly Americans. *Journal of Health and Social Behavior, 27,* 209.

IV THE INTEGRATION OF BIOLOGICAL AND SOCIAL EXPLANATIONS

10 The Twain Meet: Empirical Explanations of Sex Differences in Health and Mortality

Lois M. Verbrugge

Although men have higher mortality rates in the U.S. and other developed societies, women have higher rates of morbidity and therapeutic care. This apparent contradiction unravels quickly in analyses of detailed health statistics: The data show that women have higher rates of acute illnesses and most nonfatal chronic conditions; but men have higher prevalence rates of the leading fatal conditions, which parallels their higher mortality. These facts make the sex differentials in morbidity and mortality more compatible, but still leave unanswered the question of why those sex differences exist at all.

This chapter offers some concrete answers for women's morbidity and more active health care. We begin with a brief review of the differences in physical health and hypotheses about these differences. Using health diaries and interviews from a population-based sample

Data collection for the Health in Detroit Study was funded by the Center for Epidemiologic Studies, National Institute of Mental Health (R01 MH29478). A Biomedical Research Support Grant (Vice President for Research, The University of Michigan) provided funds for this analysis. A Research Career Development Award from the National Institute of Child Health and Human Development (K04 HD00441) facilitated the work. The author thanks Alice C. Yan for computing assistance and colleagues for comments on earlier versions. This conceptual framework and empirical data were presented in part, at the NIA Conference on Gender and Longevity, Bethesda, MD, 1987, and also appear in the *Journal of Health and Social Behavior, 30,* 282–304 (1989).

(Health in Detroit Study), we examine sex differences in daily and longer-run health, and how well acquired health risks, attitudes about illness and health care, and health reporting tendencies explain them. Starting with bivariate analyses, we report sex differences in health and the hypothesized risk factors. Multiple regression procedures then show how controlling for the hypothesized risks alters sex differences in health. We discuss particular social risks that prompt poorer health among women, and how these may mask an underlying male disadvantage. We conclude by integrating the empirical results with recent analyses of male excess mortality and arrive at a strong inference about the importance of biological factors for male's ultimate disadvantage.

The term "sex" will be used in its demographic sense, simply to designate the two population groups of interest, men and women. "Health" is a compact term that encompasses both morbidity (health status) and health behavior.

SEX DIFFERENCES IN HEALTH

Health surveys in the United States repeatedly find that women have higher overall rates of physical illness, disability days, physician visits, and prescription and nonprescription drug use than men. For the great majority of population health indicators, women's rates exceed men's. The exceptions are higher male rates for sensory/structural impairments, life-threatening chronic diseases, and long-term major disability due to chronic conditions. Young men (ages 17 to 44) have higher injury rates than young women; but for people ages 65+, women's injury rates are higher. These sex differences are reviewed extensively in (Hing, Kovar, & Rice, 1983; Nathanson, 1977; Verbrugge, 1976a, 1976b, 1982a, 1985a; Verbrugge & Wingard, 1987; Wingard, 1984; Waldron, 1982).

A close look at the health data reveals that women are more frequently sick in the short run, with higher rates of daily symptoms and higher incidence rates for acute (transient) illnesses. Over the long run, women have higher prevalence rates for numerous nonfatal chronic conditions such as arthritis, chronic sinusitis, and digestive conditions (Vergrugge, 1985a, 1989). These cause abundant symptoms, disability, and medical care, but not death. By contrast, men have higher prevalence rates of ischemic heart disease, atherosclerosis, emphysema, and other fatal conditions.[1] Men's higher mortality rates are an understandable consequence.

THEORETICAL EXPLANATIONS

Five types of reasons have been proposed to account for sex differences in health: (1) Biological risks; these are intrinsic differences between males and females based on their genes or hormones, which confer differential risks of morbidity. (2) Acquired risks; these are risks of illness and injury encountered in work and leisure activities, life-style and health habits, psychological distress, and other aspects of a person's social milieu. (3) Psychosocial aspects of symptoms and care; this is how people perceive symptoms, assess their severity, decide what to do to relieve or cure health problems, and their ability to take desired actions. (This set is commonly called "illness behavior" in medical sociology; Mechanic, 1962, 1978.) (4) Health reporting behavior; this is how people talk about their symptoms to others, including interviewers. (5) Prior health care and caretakers; this is how therapeutic actions chosen by oneself or by a health professional influence the course of current diseases and the future onset of new ones.

Of these five factors, two are widely thought by scientists to disfavor men with respect to health and longevity: biological risks and (less) prior care. Two are thought to boost women's morbidity experiences and reports: psychosocial aspects and health reporting behavior. Acquired risks are considered a mix: Some key life-style behaviors (smoking, alcohol consumption, and occupational hazards) are more common for men, giving them higher long-term risks; but other life-style behaviors (less strenuous leisure activity, overweight, stresses and unhappiness, and role pressures) are believed to put females at higher risk. Specific hypotheses have been spelled out amply elsewhere (Mechanic, 1976; Nathanson, 1975, 1977; Verbrugge, 1976b, 1979, 1985a).

This analysis will consider hypotheses for three domains: acquired risks, psychosocial aspects, and (to a limited extent) health reporting behavior. It cannot test how health care influences future health because the interview data are cross-sectional and the prospective data (health diaries) cover too short a time period. It also does not test directly the impact of biological risks as these are very difficult to measure in a survey (or any other) setting.

RESEARCH STRATEGIES

Multivariate research on sex differences has tackled two questions: "Do men and women differ in their levels of risk factors, and does this account for their health differences?" and "Do equivalent risk factors have a stronger impact on one sex's health than the other's?" The first question concerns risk exposure, and the second, risk responsiveness. Statistically, they are measured by additive (main) and interaction effects, respectively.

The *risk exposure* approach is typical in research on sex differences in physical health and mortality. Analyses center on how the differences in men's and women's lives and environments cause one sex to have more ailments and health care. Studies to date point toward role statuses, role satisfaction, stressors, and health attitudes as powerful factors behind sex differences in health. Specifically, women's lesser employment, lower levels of satisfaction, higher perceived stress, and positive predispositions toward health care are pertinent. The main reason for women's higher rates of health behavior is their higher morbidity (reproductive conditions included or not).

The *risk responsiveness* approach has been favored in research on sex differences in mental health, in which a prominent issue has been reactions to stress and other disruptions. Factors most often implicated in women's poorer mental health are role statuses (main effects) and higher responsiveness to stress.

Two footnotes expand the summaries above for physical and mental health.[2,3] This article will concentrate on the issue of risk exposure, in line with other research on physical health.[4]

DATA SOURCE

Data for the analyses here come from the Health in Detroit Study, a survey of white adults (ages 18+) residing in the Detroit metropolitan area in Fall 1978. A multistage probability sample of households was selected (institutional and military sites excluded). In each household, one adult was chosen as the study respondent by a random procedure. An initial interview was conducted in-person on health and psychosocial attributes. Then respondents kept Daily Health Records (a health diary) for 6 weeks. Questions on symptoms, health actions, mood, and special events were answered each day. At the end of the diary period, a brief termination interview was conducted by telephone.[5]

There are 714 respondents (302 men, 412 women) who completed an initial interview (II). Among them, 589 (243 men, 346 women) kept at least one week of Daily Health Records (DHR). This analysis draws on both the interview and diary information. The diary variables are aggregated counts over the 6-week period. Information for each diary-keeper is standardized to a 6-week period; this adjusts for truncated diaries due to dropout (Verbrugge, 1984).

Variables

The analysis has a large scope, involving 67 dependent variables and initially 40 predictors (named in Appendix 1).[6] We considered this the best way to obtain general conclusions about the causes of sex differences, which are durable and replicable.

The *dependent variables* (n = 67) span health status and behavior in the long and short run. The majority have significant sex differences (n = 45, $p \leq .05$). Whenever possible, parallel items in the interview and diary were selected (e.g., bed days in past year and in 6 weeks). Altogether, 34 variables from the initial interview were used (23 health status, 11 health behavior), and 33 from the Daily Health Records (20 health status, 13 health behavior).

Predictor variables are in 8 conceptual groups. Lifestyle, Roles, Stress, and Socioeconomic pertain to acquired risks. Health Attitudes, Psychological, and Structural/Enabling refer to psychosocial aspects. There are no subgroups for Health Reporting Behavior. (See Appendix 1 for details.) The predictors are all plausible candidates for explaining sex differences in health, as they are thought to differ by sex and also be associated with health. (The last predictor, health reporting behavior, affects reports not health itself).

Three *other independent variables* are used: (1) Age is strongly associated with health, a reflection of accumulated risks up to current age (social) and of gradual decline in physiological resistance and resilience with age (biological). By controlling for age, we can see more clearly how social factors, on their own, propel poor health and therapeutic care; (2) Morbidity enters as a control in equations for health behaviors, so we can see how predictors affect care independent of their effects on morbidity itself; and (3) Sex is the central predictor, whose effect is watched as other predictors are statistically controlled.

Figure 10.1 portrays the key concepts and their theoretical positions. Our empirical analyses are extensive and the results cannot be shown in full detail; readers are welcome to contact the author for any not shown in subsequent sections (including correlation matrices for models).

HYPOTHESES FOR THIS ANALYSIS

The following hypotheses are based on our extensive review of literature in this area.

Figure 10.1 Key concepts for this analysis.

Hypothesized Risk Factors
  Acquired Risks
    Lifestyle
    Roles
    Stress
    Socioeconomic
  Psychosocial Aspects
    Health Attitudes
    Psychological
    Structural/Enabling
  Health Reporting Behavior
Other Independent Variables
  Age
  Morbidity
  Sex
Dependent Variables
  Health Status
  Health Behavior

Sex Differences in Health

We anticipate that women's excess for health problems and health care is larger for daily health than for broad time spans (such as "in the past year"). This hypothesis stems from prior surveys that suggest sex differences are bigger for "minor" than "major" ailments. Because daily health includes symptoms of all severity levels, especially minor ones, we may find the largest sex differences there.

Sex Differences in Predictors

On average, we expect these differences between men and women: Men's life-styles include more smoking, alcohol consumption, and hazards; but men also have moderate sleep, less overweight, and more physical activity than women. Men are more often employed and married. Basic parental responsibility as indicated by number of children and overall role satisfaction are similar for the sexes. Women report more stress and unhappiness, and their socioeconomic status is lower than men's. We expect women to have stronger health predispositions than men (higher valuation of health, stronger belief in merits of restricted activity, etc.). Women feel less mastery and self-esteem in life overall. They have fewer fixed time constraints (due largely to less job participation) than men. They more often have a regular physician; other structural/enabling characteristics may not differ much by sex. Women are more enthusiastic about reporting their health in surveys.

Risk Factors for Poor Health

Several risk factors for poor health are hypothesized:

Acquired Risks

Health status is worse among people who currently smoke (and possibly those who previously smoked), drink alcohol frequently or did so regularly in the past, sleep few or many hours each day, are overweight, have little routine or strenuous physical activity, and are exposed to hazards at job or home. Employment and marriage are linked to good health status. Parental responsibilities have a curvilinear tie; people with several young children or none have worse health than those with just one child. Role attachments (employment, marriage, parenthood) reduce people's care for their symptoms. Dissatisfaction with one's main role, and all facets of stress, are associated with poor health status and more care for symptoms. Education and income are inversely related to health status. No hypotheses are stated for relationships between health behavior and life-style/socioeconomic factors.

Psychosocial Aspects

Strong health motivations increase both symptom perception and symptom care. A sturdy psychological foundation reduces symptom experience and also symptom care (people eschew the sick role). Time demands have a curvilinear link to health status; people with very low or very high constraints/pressures have higher morbidity than those with moderate ones. A monotonic pattern should appear for health behavior, with less care as time demands rise. People who have trouble cutting back on activities when ill show a preference for medical care, while those who have trouble leaving their job or home to see a physician opt more for self-care. Good access to medical care increases visits to physicians and most self-care actions as well.

Health-Reporting Behavior

Interviewers judged respondents' health-reporting behavior by several items at the end of the interview. We expect that interest in the survey and good recall about past health events increase health reports in the interview. Impatience about finishing the interview reduces them.

Explaining Sex Differences

If the hypotheses above about sex differences in predictors and risk factors are true, then: Women are at greater risk than men from almost all the social factors—most life-style items; lower role involvement; higher stress; lower socioeconomic status; health concern and attitudes; weaker psychological base; fewer time constraints; better access to a regular physician; and greater eagerness to report health problems. Men are at greater risk in just a few life-style behaviors (though these prove crucial for fatal morbidities). Because the preponderance of health risks weigh against women, we expect that controlling for predictors will typically narrow sex differences in health; that is, reduce women's disadvantage.

BIVARIATE RESULTS

We now present bivariate relations of sex with health and sex with the predictors, as a descriptive foundation for the multivariate analyses. Tables showing these sex differences are previously published (Verbrugge, 1988) and are not repeated here. Discussion of risk factors for poor health will follow the multivariate results.

Sex Differences in Health

Almost all of the health indicators show higher morbidity and health care for women (60 of 67, 90%). The majority of the female excesses are statistically significant (42 of 60, 70%, $p \leq .05$). In the discussion below, results are statistically significant (SIG, $p \leq .05$) unless noted (NS $p > .05$).

Specifically, in the interview, women rate their health poorer than men do. During the past year, they have been troubled by more chronic conditions and symptoms. The female excess appears in almost all body systems, being especially large for circulation (other than heart disease/high blood pressure; includes varicose veins and hemorrhoids), blood (mostly anemia), and nervous system (mostly migraine) conditions. Only for impairments are men's rates higher. When medical coding is applied to these self reports, results are still parallel: Women have more chronic diseases and chronic symptoms; men have more injuries with chronic outcomes.

In the short run of 6 weeks, women typically feel worse than men. They have more symptomatic days and more total health problems.

Most body systems show more symptoms among women (9 of 10, 6 SIG). Respondents named the presumed causes for their symptoms: Women have more symptoms attributed to disease and "other" reasons (overexertion, lack of sleep, etc.). Women have more symptoms at all severity levels, but especially those rated as "very serious."

In the past year, women have had more short-term disability days and also more long-term limitations (results consistent but NS). They have visited physicians for preventive care more often; the average number of curative visits is the same for men and women. Women report much greater curative and preventive drug use. Parallel sex differences appear in the diary: Women have more restricted activity days, especially bed days, more preventive medical care, and notably more drug use of all kinds in 6 weeks. Women talk with family and friends about symptoms on more days than men do.

As hypothesized, sex differences in morbidity are often larger for the short run than the long run. For example, the sex ratio (F/M) for total symptoms in 6 weeks is 1.66, compared to 1.22 for total chronic problems in past year. For disease problems in 6 weeks, the ratio is 2.01, compared to 1.36 for chronic diseases in past year. There are 11 health-status items sufficiently parallel to compare in the diaries and interviews; 7 of them show a distinctly larger female excess in the diaries. Though this evidence is not homogeneous, it does tend to show that women are much more bothered by daily physical symptoms than men, and the gap narrows for longer-run problems. The diary excess should not be attributed solely to "minor" problems since daily symptoms are a mix of acute and chronic types, varying in severity. Simple assertions that interviews measure "major" health problems, and diaries "minor" ones, should be abandoned.

Sex Differences in Predictors

Our hypotheses about sex differences in acquired risks, psychosocial aspects, and health reporting behavior are largely supported by the data. In the following discussion, differences are statistically significant ($p \leqslant .05$) unless noted.

Acquired Risks

(a) *Lifestyle:* men are significantly more likely to have a history of smoking, and they are more likely (but NS) to currently smoke. Men currently drink alcohol, and do so frequently, more than women. Men tend to sleep few hours ($\leqslant 6$) and women many ($9+$) in a 24-hour period. The men *in this study* tend toward overweight slightly more than women. (The sleep and weight results are contrary to hypothesis.) Women have far less strenuous (aerobic) leisure activity each week. Men report more hazards in their daily environments, largely located at their job sites.

(b) *Roles:* women are less likely than men to be currently employed or currently married (more are previously married). There is no significant difference in basic parental responsibility (number of own preschool children at home) or in feelings about main role (job or housework) (but see Verbrugge, 1982c for subgroup differences).

(c) *Stress:* recent stress is higher for women than men. Other indicators of unhappiness and stress tend to be higher for women, too, but not by much (NS for general wellbeing, persistent stress, number of stressful life events in past year).

(d) *Socioeconomic:* men have higher educational attainment and higher family incomes.

Psychosocial Aspects

(a) *Health Attitudes:* attitudes routinely point in the direction of more salience and concern by women, whether the differences are statistically significant or not. The significant differences are: Women value health more than men do, and they have more responsibility to care for ill family members (indicates more attentiveness to health matters). They believe more strongly that personal actions contribute to good health, yet they feel much more vulnerable to illness. Women are more convinced than men that medical care is efficacious.

(b) *Psychological:* there are sharp sex differences here: Men feel more mastery in their lives and have higher self-esteem. Women do, however, say they try to look on the positive side of things, more than men.

(c) *Structural/Enabling:* men have more committed hours each week, but there is no difference in how time-pressured the two sexes feel. Women say it is more difficult to drop regular activities when ill to take restricted activity. Though women have a regular physician much more often, they have health insurance coverage less often than men. Men and women similarly rate their degree of knowledge about health/disease.

Health Reporting Behavior

According to interviewers, women respondents were more interested in the interview. Impatience to finish it was similar for the sexes; recall ability was judged slightly better for men (NS).

Age (Control Variable)

On average, women are a little older than men (NS), a typical situation in population-based samples.

Summary

(1) Men appear broadly advantaged by their participation in productive and personally fulfilling roles, life satisfaction and felt stress, socioeconomic status, and some life-style behaviors. They seem disadvantaged only in smoking, alcohol consumption, overweight, and recognized exposure to hazards. (2) Popular beliefs about women's health perceptions and concern receive consistent, but generally small, support. These differences should not be exaggerated; men's and women's health attitudes are really more similar than they are different. Women's psychological makeup is less robust overall. Men are deterred from health care from objective time constraints and fewer established ties to physicians, but they have less trouble taking time for care and more insurance resources to do so. (3) There are no consistent sex differences in health reporting behavior.

MULTIVARIATE RESULTS

What happens to sex differences if predictors are controlled; that is, made statistically similar for men and women? Do our predictors suffice to explain women's higher morbidity and health care?

The multivariate analyses use multiple regression procedures. All dependent variables are interval-scaled,[7] and most of the independent variables are interval-scaled (categorical ones treated as dummy variables, ordinal ones as interval or dummy depending on hypotheses about their effects).

A sequence of regressions is estimated. We begin with the *observed sex difference:* Y = f[Sex] (Model I). *Controls* are added at the next stage: Y = f[Sex, Age] (Model II) for health status, and Y = f[Sex, Age, Morbidity] (Model IIA) for health behaviors. How each *predictor group* ($n = 8$) influences the sex difference is then studied: Y = f[Sex, Controls, Predictor Group i] (Model III). Finally, a *complete* model with all predictors is estimated: Y = f[Sex, Controls, All X] (Model IV).

To assess how the sex difference changes, we look at the significance, direction, and sign of the sex coefficient. Specifically, we consider (1) whether significant ($p \leq .05$, SIG) differences become nonsignificant ($p > .05$, NS), or vice versa; (2) the usual direction of shifts—toward smaller, larger, or even reversed effects; and (3) the size of shifts as different predictors enter. Though these are interrelated facets of the results, they give distinct perspectives. Table 10.1 summarizes the changes in the sex differences for each perspective; the text below will guide readers through it. (Detailed results for selected health variables are found in Verbrugge, 1988).

Significance Level

Of the 67 dependent variables, 45 have a *significant* ($p \leq .05$) observed sex difference. What happens to significance level from Model I to IV, as more predictors are entered? (See Table 10.1 top panel, left side.) For health status (HS): Age (Model II) reduces the sex differences just a little and they remain significant. When predictor groups are controlled one by one (Model III), sex differences narrow considerably and become nonsignificant. This occurs more often in the interview than the diary. When all predictors are included (Model IV), most of the sex differences disappear statistically. For health behavior (HB): Sex differences start to disappear when morbidity is controlled (Model IIA), especially in the diaries. After that point, predictor groups do not push sex differences much farther. The full array of predictors is, however, sufficient to make most of them ultimately disappear.

Consider the *nonsignificant* ($n = 22$) sex differences (Table 10.1 top panel, right side). If suppressors are operating to make some sex differences "abnormally" small, we may find some shifts from NS to SIG in the multivariate setting. But almost none occur; most (20) of the differences remain NS in the final model. Thus, suppressors are not a powerful or common aspect of sex differences in real-life rates.

Direction

Now we concentrate on the direction of changes, comparing Model I to Model IV (Table 10.1 second panel).

Among the 45 significant differences, 42 show a female excess and 3 a male excess. Virtually all of the *female excesses* (41) *diminish* in the presence of predictors (38 become NS). Strikingly, 6 of the items reverse their sign to reveal an ultimate male disadvantage. These new male excesses are NS, but nonetheless remarkable and a complete surprise. They are: interview data, total number of chronic problems, number of chronic symptoms, and presence of heart trouble in past year; for the diary data, number of restricted activity days, reduced chores days, and days with curative medical visits. Of the 3 *male excesses,* 2 become *larger* than originally. They are: interview data, number of injuries with chronic outcomes and number of impairments from old accident/injury.

Among the 22 nonsignificant differences, 18 have a female excess and 4 a male one. Almost all the *female excesses* (14) *reverse* to reveal a male excess. Two from the interview data become significant: job limitations and all limitations due to health. The others are: HS(II): days ill in past 2 weeks, heart trouble ever, any chronic musculoskeletal condition, allergies, chronic eye/ear disease; HS(DHR): number of musculoskeletal symptoms; HS(II): restricted activity days in past 2 weeks, same in past year, bed days in past year, visits to medical doctor in past year; HB(DHR): number of preventive drugs, number of prescription drugs. Of the 4 *male excesses,* 3 *expand* to show a larger male disadvantage than before, but remain NS. They are: curative medical visits in past year, number of skin symptoms, and number of symptoms due to injury.

Summing up, in Table 10.1 we have *boxed* the changes that favor females; stated otherwise, they disfavor males. These are female excesses that narrow or even reverse to a male excess, and male excesses that expand or remain stable. The *unboxed* categories have the opposite interpretation; they favor males and disfavor females. The data yield 63 circled items and only 4 uncircled ones. Thus, statistically making men and women similar in their risks slowly removes females' disadvantage; in other words, it works against men.

Especially striking are the 20 items (30% of 67) that begin with a female excess and reverse to a male one. They are not haphazard events, but instead appear precisely in items where a fundamental male disadvantage is commonly assumed, and the observed female one thus seems odd: presence of heart disease, total number of chronic problems, number of chronic symptoms (usually undiagnosed conditions), musculoskeletal conditions and symptoms,[8] disability days from health problems, and long-term limitations. The expansion of initial male excesses for injuries and impairments also aligns with those assumptions. Even some important health care items reverse; final models show higher rates among men for curative medical care visits and prescription drug use. The reversals seldom reach statistical significance. Their importance lies in their *frequency* (30%), *reasonableness* (items that have good interpretation, admittedly post hoc), and *consistency* (arising in both the interview and diaries). These three features suggest that something more than chance is operating for the male excesses.

Overall, the results in this section signal reduction of the female disadvantage, and potential exposure of a male disadvantage in

Table 10.1 Accounting for Sex Differences in Health[a]

How significance level of sex coefficient changes

	Significant Sex Differences				Nonsignificant Sex Differences			
	II:HS	DHR:HS	II:HB	DHR:HB	II:HS	DHR:HS	II:HB	DHR:HB
N =	15	15	4	11	8	5	7	2
	No. *NS* by model stated at left				No. *SIG* by model stated at left			
II: Age	1	0	0	0	0	0	0	0
IIA: Age, morbidity	—	—	1	7	—	—	0	0
III: Predictor group								
Lifestyle	3	2	3	7	0	1	0	0
Roles	8	4	2	7	0	1	4	0
Stress	7	2	1	7	0	1	0	0
Socioeconomic	3	2	1	7	0	1	0	0
Health Attitudes	11	4	2	8	0	0	0	0
Psychological	4	1	1	7	0	1	0	0
Structural/Enabling	6	5	2	9	0	0	2	0
Reporting	2	0	1	7	0	0	0	0
IV: All Predictors	12	12	3	10	0	0	2	0

How direction of sex coefficient changes

Shifts in Direction from Model I to Full Model (IV)

	Initial Female Excess		Initial Male Excess	
	HS	HB	HS	HB
SIG N =	27	15	(SIG) 3	0
Stays F but smaller / Stays M but smaller	24	11	1	—
Flips to M / Flips to F	3	3	0	—
Becomes bigger F / Becomes bigger M	0	0	2	—
No change	0	1	0	—
NS N =	10	8	(NS) 3	1
Stays F but smaller / Stays M but smaller	3	0	1	0
Flips to M / Flips to F	6	8	0	0
Becomes bigger F / Becomes bigger M	0	0	2	1
No change	1	0	0	0

Table 10.1 (continued)

How size of sex coefficient changes
SIG differences with female excess[b]

	Average percent decline in coefficient (Model I to model stated at left)[c]			
N=	II:HS 6	DHR:HS 9	II:HB 4	DHR:HB 11
II: Age	11%	1%	8%	2%
IIA: Age, morbidity	—	—	28	56
III: Predictor group				
Lifestyle	-10^d	-1	37 (9)[e]	68 (12)
Roles	54	24	41 (13)	65 (9)
Stress	44	29	30 (2)	56 (0)
Socioeconomic	31	6	25 (-3)	59 (3)
Health Attitudes	77	29	53 (25)	62 (6)
Psychological	27	9	29 (1)	58 (2)
Structural/Enabling	36	23	38 (10)	69 (13)
Reporting	27	9	30 (2)	57 (1)
IV: All Predictors	94	63	70	76

— Inap. for Panels 1 and 3, dash means the model is Inap and thus not estimated. For Panel 2, dash means no sex differences in the overall grouping existsn.
[a] Equations for Models I, II, IIA, III, and IV are in the text.
[b] For HS, only general items are considered, not the specific condition items. For HB, all available items are considered.
[c] A reversal from female to male excess is counted as 100%, not more.
[d] A minus sign means the coefficient is *larger* than Model I by that percentage.
[e] In ( ), % decline from Model IIA to the model stated at far left.

KEY: II, Initial Interview; SIG, $p \leq .05$; DHR, Daily Health Records; NS, $p > .05$; HS, Health status; M, Male; HB, Health behavior; F, Female.

aspects relevant to long-term fatal morbidity. The important point is the consistent story these changes tell, not simply their level of statistical significance.

Size

When predictors are entered, sex differences narrow for almost all dependent variables (60 of 67). But certain predictor groups do this job better than others. Comparing Model III with Models I and II, we can see the relative importance of conceptual groups. We discuss here their ability to explain sex differences for the principal health items, those showing a significant female excess at the outset.

For *health status* items, Health Attitudes explain the female excess best, followed by Roles and Stress (Table 10.1 third panel). Structural/Enabling takes middle rank; the other groups (Socioeconomic, Psychological, Reporting) are lower. The surprise is Lifestyle; its negative sign means that controlling for such risks often elevates the female excess. We noted earlier that some lifestyle factors disfavor men, and others women; altogether, the first aspect dominates. Expansion of the sex difference is a genuine suppressor effect; it appears often for Lifestyle but is small and entirely offset by other predictors in larger models (IV). This means that if women had certain lifestyle habits like men's (especially current and past smoking, and hazardous exposures), their health would worsen and real-world sex differences would be even larger.

For *health behavior* items, Morbidity is the main force behind actions. Its importance is especially clear in the prospective (diary) data, which give a better view of causal links between symptoms and care than the interview does. For the diary, Structural/Enabling items rank after Morbidity. For the interview, Health Attitudes rank next in power, then Roles; the other groups are about equal. Lifestyle factors here work to reduce the female excess.

Summary

Controlling for a wide array of social factors makes sex differences in health narrow and often vanish statistically. Thus, differences in men's and women's social exposures are largely responsible for the different levels of morbidity they experience. (By social exposure, we mean the domains of acquired risks, psychosocial aspects, and health-reporting behavior.)

Beyond this, the data show that initial female excesses often reverse to reveal male ones in the final model. These are consistent, albeit numerically small, signs of an underlying health disadvantage for men.

RISK FACTORS AND THE SEX AT RISK

Which personal characteristics increase morbidity and therapeutic efforts the most? And which specific risk factors drive sex differences the most? We present here condensed results on both questions.

Principal Risks

The most important risk factors for poor *health status* in the Detroit study are older age, current smoking, nonemployment, role dissatisfaction and overall stress, low mastery, low and (to a smaller degree) high time constraints, and a sense of vulnerability to illness. In a second tier of importance are little strenuous leisure activity, nonmarriage, high family health care responsibility, and low or high time pressures. Past regular drinking is tied to poor health; both causation and selection (poor health forces people to stop drinking) are implicated. Reporting effects do exist; interest in the study boosts reports, mostly in the interview. Typically, these effects appear in both the interview and diaries. This gives grist to our thinking about them in causal terms, because the predictors precede in time the health events for the diary data.

Morbidity is the strongest propeller of *health care*. Beyond its impact, factors that especially push ill people to care for their problems are older age, nonemployment, stress of all kinds, low and (to a smaller degree) high time constraints, and positive predispositions about the sick role. Other important, less strong propellers are: low income, high valuation of health, freedom from responsibility for family health care, illness vulnerability, health fatalism, low self-esteem, low time pressures, health insurance, having a regular physician, and medical sophistication. These are all potentially causal relations as the reverse routes usually make little sense, and because the associations appear for prospective as well as retrospective health data.

Table 10.2 presents these net effects in a more visual manner. It condenses the regression results greatly, and we recommend that readers rely on the narrative above and refer to the table only for details. Virtually all stated hypotheses about risk factors for poor health are confirmed; a footnote indicates the principal exceptions.[9]

The data really contain three time perspectives: the short run of symptoms in 6 weeks, the middle run of health events during the past year, and the long run of having chronic problems and major disability from them. Our analyses show that risk factors found for one time frame reappear in the others. (Their patterns of influence are usually the same, and R^2 for comparable items are similar.) Nothing forces such parallels to happen, so they must be meaningful.

The broad similarities reflect, we believe, the continuity of causal processes in daily, yearly, and lifelong health. Going in one causal direction: High levels of acute or chronic symptoms add up to poor health on an annual basis and can lower resistance to new chronic conditions. Going in the other: Factors that cause chronic conditions to cross a diagnostic threshold also cause them to progress year by year, and to flare up in daily life. We think the strongest conclusion here pertains to the diaries: Daily symptoms are not random events at all, but are driven by the same factors and processes that cumulate into long-term health problems.

Risks that Drive Sex Differences

To be powerful in explaining sex differences, a predictor must not only be strongly related to health, but also differ in its frequency among men and women. By reviewing the detailed results for both aspects, we locate specific reasons for women's excess morbidity and health care. (Table 10.2 shows the results; degree of importance is conveyed in the Sex at Risk columns by bold upper case (strongest), plain upper case, and lower case (weakest) letters. For the moment, ignore whether the letter signifies male or female.)

Factors that account most strongly for sex differences in health status are: strenuous leisure activity, employment status, acute stress, illness vulnerability, and time constraints (and close behind, interest in survey). For health behavior, they are: morbidity and time constraints (and close behind, employment status).[10]

Impressively, the strongest risk factors (noted in the previous section) also tend to be the ones that drive sex differences most. In other words, aspects of social life that influence health most are also aspects that differ appreciably for men and women. This pairing of high risk with differential exposure makes for some very large differences in real-life health experiences of the two sexes.

The Sex at Risk

Table 10.2 shows which sex is at risk of poor health from each predictor (see letters designating male and female in the Sex at Risk columns). Most risks—whether strong or weak—are attached to females; strong ones are uniformly feminine. Contemporary life puts women, not men,

Table 10.2 Risk Factors and The Sex at Risk
(Positive (+) net effect means worse health status or more health behavior)

	Health status				Health behavior			
	Net Effect[a]		Sex at Risk[b]		Net Effect		Sex at Risk	
	II	DHR	II	DHR	II	DHR	II	DHR
Controls								
AGE	+***	·	F	F	+NS	+**	f	f
MORBIDITY		+**		F	+***	+***	F	F
Lifestyle								
SMOKE-curr	+*	+NS [c]	M	M	-NS	-NS	f	f
-past	+NS	+NS			-NS	·		
-never	-							
DRINK-curr fq	-NS	+NS [d]			+NS	+NS	m	
-curr infq				f	-NS	-NS	f	
-past reg	+NS	+**			·	+*		
-past rare		+NS			+NS	+NS		
-never	-NS	+*			·	·		
SLEEP-6 hrs. or less	+NS	·	m		·	-NS		f
-7-8	-							
-9+	-NS	-NS		·	·	+NS		
RELWGT	-NS	·	f		+NS	+NS	m	m
PHYSACTV	-NS	+NS	f	m	-NS	·	f	· M
STRENACTV	-NS	-NS	F	F		+NS		
HAZARDS	+NS	·	M	·	·	·	·	·

	1	2	3	4	5	6	7	8
Roles								
EMPL	f	F	− NS	− **	F	F	− *	− NS
MARR-curr								
-previous			+ NS				+ NS	+ NS
-never			+ NS				+ NS	+ NS
YOUNGCHD-0								
-1	f	m	− NS	− NS	m		·	− NS
-2+			− NS	+ NS			+	·
ROLEFEEL			·	+ NS	F	F	− **	− *
Stress								
GWB	F	F	− *	− ***	F	F	− *	− *
ACUTESTRESS	F		+ NS	+ NS	F	F	+ **	+ ***
CHRONICSTRESS	f	f	+ NS	+ NS	f	f	+ NS	+ NS
LIFEEVENTS	f	F	+ NS	+ **	F	F	+ **	+ **
Socioeconomic								
EDUC			·	− NS	M	F	− NS	− NS
FAMINCOME	F	F	− NS	− NS	·	F	+ NS	+ NS
Health attitudes								
VALUE	f	f	+ NS	+ NS	f	m	− NS	− NS
HLTHRESP	M	M	− NS	− NS	F	F	+ NS	+ NS
IFCUTDOWN	f	F	+ NS	+ ***			+ *	+ NS
IFSEEKCARE			− NS	− NS	M		− NS	− *
POSHEALTH	F	·	+ NS	·	F	F	+ NS	+ ***
SIGNS	m		·	+ NS	m	m	·	− *
VULNERABLE	F	F	+ NS	+ *	F	F	+ ***	+ NS
HLC/CHANCE	f	f	+ NS	+ NS	f	f	+ NS	+ NS
EFFIC/RESTACT	f	f	+ NS	+ NS			+ ***	+ NS
EFFIC/MDADV	·	·	·	·	·		·	·

Table 10.2 (continued)

Psychological								
MASTERY	– *	– NS	F	f	·	+ NS	·	m
SELFESTEEM	·	+ NS	·	M	– NS	– NS	f	f
POSITIVESIDE	·	·	·	·	·	·	·	·
Structural/enabling								
RUSHED-never								
-rarely	– NS	– NS			+ NS			
-sometimes	+ NS	· NS			+ NS			
-often	+ NS	– NS			– NS	– NS	·	·
-always	+ *	– NS			– NS	– NS	·	·
HOURS-low	+ NS	+ NS [e]	F	F	·	·	f	f
-medium	·	·			– NS	– NS		
-high	+ NS	· NS	F					
HOURS(linear)	– **	– NS	F	Fg	*	**	F	Fg
(squared)	+ **	+ NS			+	+		
DIFFIC/RESTACT		+ NS [h]						f
DIFFIC/GOTOMD		– NS					m	m
IFINSURED		+ NS			+ NS	+ NS	F	m
REGULAR		+ NS			+ NS	+ NS	f	F
KNOW		+ NS			+ NS	+ NS		f
Health reporting								
INTEREST	+ ***	+ NS	F	F	– NS	+ NS	·	F
IMPATIENCE	+ NS	– NS	·	·	– NS	+ *	·	·
RECALL	– **	– **	F	F	·	·	f	·

— Excluded dummy.

a $b_{x.y.net}$. Consistent results from Model IV are presented. Summaries are based on (1) counting rules about frequency of signs and (2) for coefficients having consistent sign, their frequency of and level of significance. The approach is conservative: A sign (+, −) means high consistency across equations; asterisks mean numerous significant effects (* mostly P≤.05, ** mostly P≤.01, *** mostly P≤.001). When signs are inconsistent, a dot is shown; significance levels are not examined.

b 'Sex at Risk' is determined by review of $r_{sex.x}$ and $b_{x.y.net}$. Sign and strength of both were examined, and rules made to determine the sex at risk and the degree of risk. There are three degrees: high (bold upper case), middle (upper case), and low (lower case). The letter M is male, F is female. The key below gives a basic view of how sex at risk is determined:

$r_{sex.x}$ (M=0, F=1)	$b_{x.y.net}$	Sex at Risk
+	+	Women
+	−	Men
−	+	Men
−	−	Women

When sex at risk cannot be determined (due to no sex difference in the predictor, no consistent x.y relationships, or competing effects for dummy variables), a dot is shown.

c II: Current smokers have worst health; DHR: past smokers do.
d II: No group has clearly worst health status; DHR: past regular drinkers do.
e Curvilinear hypotheses supported, especially for health status.
f (Skipped)
g But m for very high values.
h But — appears for restricted activity, as hypothesized.

at greater risk of daily symptoms and longer-run health troubles. Most critical are five aspects: women's lower participation in paid employment, higher levels of emotional stress, feeling of greater vulnerability to illness, fewer time constraints (associated with fewer job hours), and less strenuous physical activity each week. All of these effects are ostensibly causal.[11] Men are at high risk of morbidity in only a few ways: current and past smoking, past regular drinking, job hazards, and (for some dependent variables) very high time constraints. This study does not show men's current drinking behavior or their overweight tendency to be linked with poor health.

ILLNESS AND DEATH: THE TWAIN MEET

We now tie our results for health with comparable studies on sex differences in mortality.

Reasons for males' higher mortality rates have been discussed extensively by biological and social scientists alike. Hypotheses center on how biological and acquired risks cause fatal conditions to occur and progress; and less often, how psyche and attitudes, death reporting, and lifetime health care affect the (recorded) timing and cause of death. Reviews of hypotheses for sex mortality differences are in (Nathanson, 1984; Verbrugge, 1976a; Verbrugge and Wingard, 1987; Waldron, 1976, 1983a, 1983b, 1986; Wingard, 1984). Gradually, empirical studies that test some of these hypotheses simultaneously in a multivariate format are being conducted, asking what happens to male excess mortality when risk factors are controlled.

Three studies in California sites have assessed how differential risk exposure affects the sex mortality differential.

1. In the Alameda County Study sample, the ratio of male to female mortality rates for a 9-year period was 1.5 ($p \leqslant .001$) (1965–1974; ages 30 to 69 in 1965) (Wingard, 1982). When 16 demographic and social risk factors (queried in 1965) were controlled, the ratio *rose* to 1.7 ($p \leqslant .001$). Eight risks disfavored women, especially higher chronic morbidity in 1965 and less physical activity; only 3 weighed against men, especially cigarette smoking history and alcohol consumption. Given these opposing risks, it is not surprising that the ratio is quite stable. It ends up increasing a bit because men's risks (smoking and alcohol) are such powerful ones for mortality. Focusing on just coronary heart disease mortality, the sex difference also does not change much (2.2 to 2.3) when the 16 risk factors are controlled (Wingard, unpublished data).

2. In Rancho Bernardo, the sex ratio was 1.7 for all-cause mortality and 4.8 for ischemic heart disease (1972–1980; ages 30 to 69 at start)

(Wingard, Suarez, & Barrett-Connor, 1983). When 8 sociodemographic and physiological (e.g., blood pressure, cholesterol) risks were controlled, the overall ratio *dropped a bit* to 1.3 ($p \leq .05$), and the heart ratio narrowed to 2.4 ($p \leq .05$). Once again, more risks weighed against women (especially cholesterol), but a few powerful ones against men (cigarette smoking, high systolic blood pressure); they offset each other to produce the small net decline in the all-cause ratio. For heart mortality, statistically reducing women's cholesterol level narrows the sex ratio considerably.[12]

3. Wingard and colleagues also cite unpublished results of a San Francisco-Oakland study of 11-year mortality (1964–1975; ages 35 to 43 in 1964; study described in Friedman, Dales, & Ury, 1979). There too, controlling for 8 sociodemographic factors *scarcely changes* the sex mortality ratio for all causes, from 1.7 to 1.5. The ratio for coronary heart disease narrows from 3.2 to 2.8.

The California studies show how stable the overall sex mortality difference is when *social* factors are controlled. More risks disfavor women, a few disfavor men; the result is little net shift. Social factors also have a hard time changing the sex difference in heart mortality (Alameda County). But when *physiological* factors are included (1 item in SF-Oakland, more in Rancho Bernardo), it does narrow. Those measures are products of both biological and acquired vulnerabilities. The compelling point is that when biological components are included, though we cannot say precisely how much, the sex difference narrows.[13]

In sum, the California studies show that controlling for social risks (many against women, a few against men) does very little to the sex mortality difference. It remains, unexplained. We must either look for some quite secret, powerful social factors or else consider biological ones.

How do the mortality and morbidity analyses fit together? They are fundamentally compatible: controlling for social factors maintains the male disadvantage for mortality, and hints strongly of one for morbidity. We end up in the same place. Given that all these studies have a good compass of social factors, we are left with an old but powerful hypothesis—that biological factors are at work in men's poorer long-run health and higher mortality.

CONCLUSION

Women's excess morbidity in contemporary life is driven by social factors, especially by risks stemming from lesser employment, higher felt stress and unhappiness, stronger feelings of illness vulnerability, fewer formal time contraints (related to fewer job hours), and less physically strenuous leisure activites. If these risks are reduced—by promoting engagement in productive roles, blunting stress and fostering happiness, and encouraging aerobic activity—women are likely to feel better physically and have fewer daily symptoms and chronic health problems. The causal processes tying these risks to health are not completely spelled out in this or other empirical research, but there is strong theory and consensus that these routes exist; finding them in the Detroit prospective (diary) data is important support. Sex differences would narrow considerably, so much that we might begin to see higher morbidity rates among men, especially for overall and chronic health indicators. Real-world sex differences in morbidity and mortality would tally more closely than they now do. Further interpretations and policy implications of this analysis are considered in a companion aricle (Verbrugge, 1988).

The unveiling of a male health disadvantage is suggestive, not conclusive. It draws strength from its frequency and its presence in items pertinent to mortality. What shall we make of the "reversals" from a female to male excess? Because our predictors cover a broad territory of social causes, the explanation for this revealed disadvantage may lie elsewhere, in biological ones. (We acknowledge one other contender, prior care, which is also missing from the predictor list. If years of active health care give sizable long-term health benefits, then women benefit more; men are at risk. Equalizing or controlling for this would reduce any observed or estimated male disadvantage.)

The suggestion about a fundamental biological base for males' disadvantage is reached indirectly, rather than by overt measures of biological robustness, in studies to date. Ideally, a statistical approach to understanding the roles of biological and social risks on morbidity and mortality, and thereby sex differences, requires such measures. They are now generally absent from sociological and epidemiological research. To biologists, we social scientists ask: What are markers of intrinsic robustness? How do the markers vary within each sex, and how do their distributions differ between the sexes? How do the markers relate to subsequent disease processes? And how can they be measured in a population of males and females?

Even if we secure a combined array of social and biological risk factors, there is plenty of theoretical and empirical work ahead to model the ties between risks and health outcomes. How do biological and social risks interact with each other; how long do prior risks (habits and behaviors that people abandon or leave) operate, and how do they exacerbate current risks; how do concurrent social risks interact with each other? How do risks cumulate over a person's lifetime? And how do combinations of chronic diseases and impairments people have (comorbidity) affect timing and cause of death? Current multivariate studies use very rudimentary models of these processes.

In conclusion, what precedes death is a very dynamic array of risks drawn from far back in someone's lifetime and also near-at-hand experiences. They are added up over time and occasionally subtracted. They are derived from a biological substrate of original credits and debits, and from the overlay of lifetime exposures. Biology is not a minor theme; in fact, social science and epidemiologic studies end up peering strongly in that direction. Yet the vulnerabilities and resistances that males and females typically receive at conception, and how aging processes and social exposures alter the size and character of one's given robustness are not known. The single greatest need in population studies of sex differences in health and mortality is operational measures of that biological substrate.

NOTES

1. Several fatal conditions show slightly higher rates for females in self-report data, but this is negligible compared to their excess for nonfatal ones.

2. A review of research on sex differences in physical health: Having fewer role obligations does not account for women's higher rates of *health problems* (acute and chronic indicators), but they do explain women's greater likelihood of *cutting down activities* and *staying longer in bed* when ill (Marcus & Seeman, 1981a; Marcus, Seeman, & Telesky, 1983). This comes about through less employment; greater (average) time flexibility for women allows them to take more care for illness. Less employment is also a key reason why women make more *doctor visits* for chronic problems (Marcus & Siegel, 1982).

Mental distress and nurturant role obligations for one's family apparently underlie poorer *self-rated health* and more *restricted activity* for women, especially married ones (Gove & Huges, 1979; see comments by Marcus & Seeman, 1981b; Mechanic, 1980; Verbrugge, 1980a).

Preeminent reasons for women's higher *outpatient visit* rates are their larger number of chronic conditions and also pregnancy/ childbirth events (Cleary, Mechanic, & Greenley, 1982). Help-seeking tendencies also figure, though less strongly.

Another study concurs that symptom experience is the main reason behind women's higher medical care contact rates (Hibbard & Pope,

1983). Beyond morbidity, health interest and concern (more common among women) helps explain it. That attitude also has a differential impact, prompting care greatly for women but only slightly for men. Hibbard and Pope (1986) then split up medical visits by type (chronic disease, trauma, etc.). Sex differences in visit rates are largest for the most discretionary and mild problems, and symptom experience and health interest/concern are stronger predictors for such visits than other types. These results pinpoint key components of women's overall higher utilization and buttress the named predictors' importance.

Higher morbidity is a key reason for women's higher use and procurement of *prescription and nonprescription drugs* (Bush & Osterweis, 1978; Verbrugge, 1982b). Controlling for morbidity reduces sex differences greatly, especially for prescription items. Fuller insight comes from taking reproductive and sex-specific conditions into account. Removing from analysis women who had those conditions in the study period, and also excluding drug categories typically used for female-specific conditions for the remaining respondents, virtually eliminates sex differences in prescription drug acquisition (Svarstad, Cleary, Mechanic, & Robers, 1987). But psychosocial factors on patients' or physicians' part cannot be waived: Physicians tend to prescribe more drugs to women for virtually all kinds of health problems, even after medical factors (such as patient age, seriousness) are controlled (Verbrugge & Steiner, 1981, 1985). Also, women's acquisition of psychotropic drugs is influenced by role responsibilities, family structure, and stressful events among family members (after controlling for sociodemographic, health, and access factors), whereas men's is not (Cafferata, Kasper, & Bernstein, 1983).

Men and women do not differ much in their pace of medical care for very serious diseases or common daily symptoms: The time interval from first noticing cancer symptoms to disease diagnosis is similar for men and women; thus, men do not delay care for this important disease (Marshall, Gregorio, & Walsh, 1982). That time interval can be split further to see patient delay (symptom onset to *first medical contact*) and diagnositc delay (contact to *diagnosis*). A study of colorectal cancers finds that women delay seeking care more than men for rectal cancer, and they experience more diagnostic delay for colon cancer (Marshall & Funch, 1986). No psychosocial reasons could be found for the first result; both physician and patient factors are implicated in the second. For symptoms of everyday life, men and women take actions at similar paces for respiratory problems and transient musculoskeletal ones (injury/overexertion); but men do respond more for musculoskeletal disease (arthritis) symptoms, possibly because such symptoms are less familiar intrusions for them than for women (Verbrugge & Ascione, 1987). Chronic knee pain is also a common symptom, slightly more prevalent among women than men. Yet men with arthritis (X-ray evidence) report more pain than comparable women (Davis, 1981). This occurs at all severity grades, and also whether people know the diagnosis or not. The reason for men's reporting is unknown, but may lie in different arthritis origins for the sexes (a medical reason) or different reactions to such pain (a psychosocial one).

Men and women differ notably in role changes for serious diseases: Among heart surgery patients, men were more likely to *return to their work* within a year than women (Brown & Rawlinson, 1977; sizable difference is NS because of small sample). (Work is the person's pre-surgery instrumental role, either job or housework.) The forces helping return to work differed: Shortness of time off work before surgery speeded men's return, while having few postoperative physical symptoms speeded women's. In another study, people hospitalized for coronary heart disease symptoms were followed for two years (Chirikos & Nickel, 1984). Of those employed before the event, men were more likely to return to work than women. Key reasons for women's not doing so were older average age and lower income (labor force withdrawal is greater for low income groups); these are exposure effects. There are also response effects; having activity limitations after the coronary event deterred women from returning to work more than it did men. This result aligns closely with the first study mentioned in this paragraph.

Focusing on a critical outcome of illness and injury, *work disability:* Having chronic symptoms and activity limitations causes work disability (restrictions in amount or kind of market work) more readily among women than men (Chirikos & Nestel, 1984). This mirrors the disease-specific results above. Moreover, women with health problems (measured by an index of symptoms and limitations, or by work disability itself) are more likely to drop out of the labor force altogether than men. Or if they do stay in it, women reduce their annual work hours more. This is strongly true for black women. But white women often accommodate health problems by changing work tasks or jobs, and even by increasing work hours (at lower wages than before). Thus, the negative impact of poor health on their economic activity is sometimes smaller than for counterpart white men (Chirikos & Nestel, 1982, 1985).

3. A review of research on sex differences in mental health:

Higher *depression* among women is influenced by less involvement in employment and marriage roles, and also to lower education, lower income, and worse physical health (Aneshensel, Frerichs, & Clark, 1981; Gore & Mangione, 1983). Having children at home increases depression for women (employed or not in Aneshensel et al., 1981; employed only in Cleary & Mechanic, 1983), but not for men. Stress (both more exposure and more impact) helps account for women's higher *anxiety* and feelings (ever) of *impending nervous breakdown* (Depner & Kulka, 1979). Having few roles is linked with high *distress* (depression, anxiety, psychophysiological symptoms) for adults; but women's greater distress levels hinge more on their lack of certain roles, principally employment, than on their having fewer total roles (Thoits, 1986).

Women's higher level of *psychophysiological symptoms* is also due partly to exposure, partly to response. One study finds that women's greater likelihood of being previously married, nonemployed, or in low income households spurs more such symptoms (Reskin & Coverman, 1985). Another study shows that women's lower education and worse physical health are important causes of the sex differences (Gore & Mangione, 1983). The study further shows that certain roles have more impact and especially propel the differnece (negative effect of young children at home for women; positive benefits from part-time work for men). Kessler (1979) finds that sex differences in psychophysiological symptoms are due much more to how strongly stressors affect women, than to higher experience of stress among them. (The stressors are life events, low financial status, and physical symptoms.) Focusing on stressful life events, a subsequent study shows that certain types of events (those occurring to someone you care about rather than to yourself) especially affect women, and this differential impact fully explains sex differences in distress (here, psychophysiological symptoms and depression) (Kessler & McLeod, 1984). A more detailed look at event types (personal vs. network, controllable vs. uncontrollable) reconfirms that sex differences (anxiety, depression) are not due to differential exposure, but stem more from men's and women's different reactivity to certain events (Thoits, 1987).

A prime reason why women have more mental health care than men is that women more readily decide their distress symptoms constitute a significant emotional problem (Kessler, Brown, & Broman, 1981). Once that decision occurs, men and women are equally likely to decide they need professional help, and to get it.

4. Responsiveness to selected risk factors (roles, stress and stressful life events, time constraints, psychological characteristics) was also studied late in the analysis. Only two items showed marked differences in this regard: feelings about main role (dissatisfaction affects women's

health more than men's) (see also Verbrugge, 1986) and illness vulnerability (stronger effects for women). Further details are available on request.

5. For details about study design, see Verbrugge (1979, 1980b). Respondent selectivity and conditioning effects are discussed in Verbrugge (1980c, 1984); interviewed people who did not keep diaries were selective in three respects: young men (age <30), low education, and poor physical health or disabled. Field procedures are presented in Verbrugge and Depner (1981). A copy of the Daily Health Record is in Verbrugge (1984, 1985b).

6. Later in our work, we stripped the predictors to items with both strong net effects on health and significant sex differences. Twelve predictors met the criteria: SMOKE, STRENACTV, HAZARDS, EMPL, ACUTESTRESS, LIFEEVENTS, EDUC, HLTHRESP, VULNERABLE, MASTERY, HOURS & HOURSSQ, INTEREST (see Appendix 1 to translate mnemonics). Stripped models with these predictors yield substantive results very similar to the ones discussed in the text (full set of predictors). In one respect, the stripped models are different: They produce smaller amounts of change in the sex effect (coefficient), simply due to fewer variables operating on it.

7. The interview items on specific chronic conditions are dichotomous (Yes/No), some quite skewed. We chose to use OLS regression anyway to maintain a parallel approach across all dependent variables. This weakens results for the condition variables, but we will rarely note the details of their regression in the text.

8. Musculoskeletal diseases (largely arthritis) are more prevalent among women in the data set, but chronic musculoskeletal conditions due to injuries and impairments are more common for men. We are presumably seeing the emergence of the latter.

9. Contrary to hypothesis: Current alcohol consumption, overweight, and many (9+) hours of sleep are unrelated to health. Sensitivity to illness signs is associated with better health. High health responsibility and high self-esteem are linked to less therapeutic care for oneself. Good recall is associated with fewer health reports; we now think recall ability does not reflect motivation, but is instead an outcome of health experience—people with few events can remember them better.

10. These results for specific variables align with the earlier ones for predictor groups (see section on Multivariate Results): Health Attitudes are important via illness vulnerability, followed by health responsibility. Roles have power through employment and, to a smaller extent, feeling about role. Stress influences sex differences through

all its items. The Structural/Enabling factor of most importance is time constraints.

11. The healthy worker effect ("good health permits people to be employed") is also pertinent for the interview data. (See discussions in Verbrugge, 1983; Verbrugge & Madans, 1985; Waldron, 1980; Waldron, Herold, Dunn & Staum, 1982.)

12. Results differ in an analysis of coronary heart disease incidence in Framingham (Johnson, 1977).

13. One other study examines both risk exposure and responsiveness (Robbins, 1984). Mortality in Tecumseh, Michigan was studied over a 10 to 12 year period (ages 35 to 69 at outset). Medical status (4 cardiopulmonary measures) is controlled, then 3 social risks (social isolation, lack of job responsibility, bad habits; all associated with higher mortality). Men score higher on bad habits and social isolation, and women on lack of job responsibility; men suffer greater impact on mortality from bad habits and social isolation. Controlling for the social factors decreases the sex mortality difference; thus, this study does find some important social causes of higher male mortality. (The decomposition technique used makes it difficult to state precisely the relative importance of the factors on the sex mortality ratio.)

REFERENCES

Aday, L., Andersen, R., & Fleming, G. V. (1980). *Health care in the United States: Equitable for whom?* Beverly Hills, CA: Sage.

Andersen, R. (1968). A Behavioral Model of Families' Use of Health Services. Research Series, No. 25. Chicago, IL: Center for Health Administration Studies, University of Chicago.

Aneshensel, C. S., Frerichs, R. R., & Clark, V. A. (1981). Family roles and sex differences in depression. *Journal of Health and Social Behavior, 22,* 379–393.

Becker, M. H. (1974). The Health Belief Model and sick role behavior. *Health Education Monographs, 2,* 409–432.

Becker, M. H., Maiman, L. A., Kirscht, J. P., Haefner, D. P., & Drachman, R. H. (1977). The Health Belief Model and prediction of dietary compliance: A field experiment. *Journal of Health and Social Behavior, 18,* 348–366.

Brown, J. A., & Rawlinson, M. E. (1977). Sex differences in sick role rejection and in work performance following cardiac surgery. *Journal of Health and Social Behavior, 18,* 276–292.

Bush, P. J., & Osterweis, M. (1978). Pathways to medicine use. *Journal of Health and Social Behavior, 19,* 179–189.

Cafferata, G. L., Kasper, J., & Bernstein, A. (1983). Family roles, structure, and stressors in relation to sex differences in obtaining psychotropic drugs. *Journal of Health and Social Behavior, 24,* 133–143.

Chirikos, T. N., & Nestel, G. (1982). The economic consequences of poor health, by race and sex. *Proceedings of the American Statistical Association (Social Statistics Section)*, 473–477.

Chirikos, T. N., & Nestel, G. (1984). Economic determinants and consequences of self-reported work disability. *Journal of Health Economics, 3*, 117–136.

Chirikos, T. N., & Nestel, G. (1985). Further evidence on the economic effects of poor health. *Review of Economics and Statistics, 67*, 61–69.

Chirikos, T. N., & Nickel, J. L. (1984). Work disability from coronary heart disease in women. *Women and Health, 9*, 55–74.

Cleary, P. D., & Mechanic, D. (1983). Sex differences in psychological distress among married people. *Journal of Health and Social Behavior, 24*, 111–121.

Cleary, P. D., Mechanic, D., & Greenley, J. R. (1982). Sex differences in medical care utilization: An empirical investigation. *Journal of Health and Social Behavior, 23*, 106–119.

Davis, M. A. (1981). Sex differences in reporting osteoarthritis symptoms: A sociomedical approach. *Journal of Health and Social Behavior, 22*, 298–310.

Depner, C. E., & Kulka, R. (1979). Sex differences in psychological distress and use of professional help as a function of social and social-psychological factors. Paper presented at the American Sociological Association meetings.

Friedman, G. D., Dales, L. G., & Ury, H. K. (1979). Mortality in middle-aged smokers and nonsmokers. *New England Journal of Medicine, 300* (5), 213–217.

Frisancho, A. R. (1986). Anthropometric standards by frame size for the assessment of growth and nutritional status for use with the Frameter. Ann Arbor, MI: Health Products (2126 Ridge, 48104).

Gore, S., & Mangione, T. W. (1983). Social roles, sex roles and psychological distress: Additive and interactive models of sex differences. *Journal of Health and Social Behavior, 24*, 300–312.

Gove, W. R., & Hughes, M. (1979). Possible causes of the apparent sex differences in physical health: An empirical investigation. *American Sociological Review, 44*, 126–146.

Hibbard, J. H., & Pope, C. R. (1983). Gender roles, illness orientation and use of medical services. *Social Science and Medicine, 17*, 129–137.

Hibbard, J. H., & Pope, C. R. (1986). Another look at sex differences in the use of medical care: Illness orientation and the type of morbidities for which services are used. *Women and Health, 11*, 21–36.

Hing, E., Kovar, M. G., & Rice, D. P. (1983). Sex differences in health and use of medical care. *Vital and Health Statistics*, Series 3, No. 24, DHHS Publ. No. (PHS) 83-1408. Hyattsville, MD: National Center for Health Statistics.

Johnson, A. (1977). Sex differentials in coronary heart disease: The explanatory role of primary risk factors. *Journal of Health and Social Behavior, 18*, 46–54.

Kessler, R. C. (1979). Stress, social status, and psychological distress. *Journal of Health and Social Behavior, 20*, 259–272.

Kessler, R. C., Brown, R. L., & Broman, C. L. (1981). Sex differences in psychiatric help-seeking: Evidence from four large-scale surveys. *Journal of Health and Social Behavior, 22,* 49–64.

Kessler, R. C., & McLeod, J. D. (1984). Sex differences in vulnerability to undesirable live events. *American Sociological Review, 49,* 620–631.

Marcus, A. C., & Seeman, T. E. (1981a). Sex differences in reports of illness and disability: A preliminary test of the "fixed role obligations" hypothesis. *Journal of Health and Social Behavior, 22,* 174–183.

Marcus, A. C., & Seeman, T. E. (1981b). Comment on "Gove and Hughes, 1979". *American Sociological Review, 46,* 119–123.

Marcus, A. C., & Siegel, J. M. (1982). Sex differences in the use of physician services: A preliminary test of the fixed role hypothesis. *Journal of Health and Social Behavior, 23,* 186–197.

Marcus, A. C., Seeman, T. E., & Telesky, C. W. (1983). Sex differences in reports of illness and disability: A further test of the fixed role hypothesis. *Social Science and Medicine, 17,* 993–1002.

Marshal, J. R., Gregorio, D. I., & Walsh, D. (1982). Sex differences in illness behavior: Care seeking among cancer patients. *Journal of Health and Social Behavior, 23,* 197–204.

Marshall, J. R., & Funch, D. P. (1986). Gender and illness behavior among colorectal cancer patients. *Women and Health, 11,* 67–82.

Mechanic, D. (1962). The concept of illness behavior. *Journal of Chronic Diseases, 15,* 189–194.

Mechanic, D. (1976). Sex, illness behavior, and the use of health services. *Social Science and Medicine, 12B,* 207–214.

Mechanic, D. (1978). *Medical Sociology.* Second Edition. New York: Free Press.

Mechanic, D. (1980). Comment on "Gove and Hughes". *American Sociological Review, 45,* 513–514.

Nathanson, C. A. (1975). Illness and the feminine role: A theoretical review. *Social Science and Medicine, 9,* 57–62.

Nathanson C. A. (1977). Sex, illness, and medical care: A review of data, theory, and method. *Social Science and Medicine* 11:13–62.

Nathanson, C. A. (1984). Sex differences in mortality. In R. H. Turner & J. F. Short (Eds.), *Annual Review of Sociology,* Vol. 10 (pp. 191–213). Palo Alto, CA: Annual Reviews Inc.

Reskin, B. F., & Coverman, S. (1985). Sex and race in the determinants of psychophysical distress: A reappraisal of the sex-role hypothesis. *Social Forces, 63,* 1038–1059.

Robbins, C. A. (1984). *Psychosocial Sources of the Sex Differences in Mortality.* Doctoral dissertation (Sociology). Ann Arbor, MI: The University of Michigan.

Schneider, D., Appleton, L. & McLemore, T. (1979). A reason for visit classification for ambulatory care. *Vital and Health Statistics,* Series 2, No. 78. DHEW Publ. No. (PHS) 79-1352. Hyattsville, MD: National Center for Health Statistics.

Svarstad, B. L., Cleary, P. D., Mechanic, D., & Robers, P. A. (1987). Gender differences in the acquisition of prescribed drugs: An epidemiological study. *Medical Care, 25,* 1089–1098.

Thoits, P. A. (1986). Multiple identities: Examining gender and marital status differences in distress. *American Sociological Review, 51,* 259–272.

Thoits, P. A. (1987). Gender and marital status differences in control and distress: Common stress versus unique stress explanations. *Journal of Health and Social Behavior, 28,* 7–22.

Verbrugge, L. M. (1976a). Sex differentials in morbidity and mortality in the United States. *Soical Biology, 23,* 275–296.

Verbrugge, L. M. 1976b. Females and illness: Recent trends in sex differences in the United States. *Journal of Health and Social Behavior, 17,* 387–403.

Verbrugge, L. M. 1979. Female ilness rates and illness behavior: Testing hypotheses about sex differences in health. *Women and Health, 4,* 61–79.

Verbrugge, L. M. 1980a. Comment on "Gove and Hughes, 1979". *American Sociological Review, 45,* 507–513.

Verbrugge, L. M. 1980b. Health diaries. *Medical Care, 18,* 73–95.

Verbrugge, L. M. 1980c. Sensitization and fatigue in health diaries. *Proceedings of the American Statistical Association (Survey Research Methods Section),* 666–671.

Verbrugge, L. M. 1982a. Sex differentials in health. *Public Health Reports, 97,* 417–437.

Verbrugge, L. M. 1982b. Sex differences in legal drug use. *Journal of Social Issues, 38,* 59–76.

Verbrugge, L. M. 1982c. Work satisfaction and physical health. *Journal of Community Health, 7,* 262–283.

Verbrugge, L. M. 1983. Multiple roles and physical health of women and men. *Journal of Health and Social Behavior, 24,* 16–30.

Verbrugge, L. M. 1984. Health diaries—problems and solutions in study design. In C. F. Cannell & R. M. Groves (Eds.), *Health Survey Research Methods,* (pp. 171–192). Research Proceedings Series. DHHS Publ. No. (PHS) 84-3346. Rockville, MD: National Center for Health Services Research.

Verbrugge, L. M. 1985a. Gender and health: An update on hypotheses and evidence. *Journal of Health and Social Behavior, 26,* 156–182.

Verbrugge, L. M. 1985b. Triggers of symptoms and health care. *Social Science and Medicine, 20,* 855–876.

Verbrugge, L. M. 1986. Role burdens and physical health of women and men. *Women and Health, 11,* 47–77.

Verbrugge, L. M. 1988. Unveiling higher morbidity for men: The story. In M. W. Riley (Ed.), *Social structures and human lives,* Vol. 1 (pp. 138–160), *Social change and the life course.* American Sociological Association Presidential Series. Newbury Park, CA: Sage.

Verbrugge, L. M. 1990. Pathways of health and death. In R. D. Apple (Ed.), *The History of Women, Health and Medicine in America* (pp. 41–79). New York: Garland.

Verbrugge, L. M., & Ascione, F. J. (1987). Exploring the iceberg: Common symptoms and how people care for them. *Medical Care, 25,* 539–569.

Verbrugge, L. M., & Depner, C. E. (1981). Methodological analyses of Detroit health diaries. In S. Sudman (Ed.), *Health survey research methods—Third Conference* (pp. 144–158). Research Proceedings Series. DHHS Publ. No.

(PHS) 81-3268. Hyattsville, MD: National Center for Health Services Research.

Verbrugge, L. M., & Madans, J. H. (1985). Social roles and health trends of American women. *Milbank Memorial Fund Quarterly/Health and Society, 63,* 691–735.

Verbrugge, L. M., & Steiner, R. P. (1981). Physician treatment of men and women patients—sex bias or appropriate care? *Medical Care, 19,* 609–632.

Verbrugge, L. M., & Steiner, R. P. (1985). Prescribing drugs to men and women. *Health Psychology, 4,* 79–98.

Verbrugge, L. M., & Wingard, D. L. (1987). Sex differentials in health and mortality. *Women and Health, 12,* 103–145.

Waldron, I. (1976). Why do women live longer than men? *Social Science and Medicine, 10,* 349–362.

Waldron, I. (1980). Employment and women's health: An analysis of causal relationships. *International Journal of Health Services, 10,* 434–454.

Waldron, I. (1982). An analysis of causes of sex differences in mortality and morbidity. In W. R. Gove & G. R. Carpenter (Eds.), *The fundamental connection between nature and nurture* (pp. 69–115). Lexington, MA: Lexington Books.

Waldron, I. (1983a). Sex differences in human mortality: The role of genetic factors. *Social Science and Medicine, 17,* 321–333.

Waldron, I. (1983b). Sex differences in illness incidence, prognosis and mortality: Issues and evidence. *Social Science and Medicine, 17,* 1107–1123.

Waldron, I. (1986). The contribution of smoking to sex differences in mortality. *Public Health Reports, 101,* 163–173.

Waldron, I., Herold, J., Dunn, D., & Staum, R. (1982). Reciprocal effects of health and labor force participation in women—evidence from two longitudinal studies. *Journal of Occupational Medicine, 24,* 126–132.

Wallston, K. A., Wallston, B. S., & DeVellis, R. (1978). Development of the Multidimensional Health Locus of Control (MHLC) Scales. *Health Education Monographs, 6,* 160–170.

Wingard, D. L. (1982). The sex differential in mortality rates. *American Journal of Epidemiology, 115,* 205–216.

Wingard, D. L. 1984. The sex differential in morbidity, mortality, and lifestyle. In L. Breslow, J. E. Fielding, & L B. Lave. (Eds.), *Annual review of public health,* Vol. 5, (pp. 433–458). Palo Alto, CA: Annual Reviews Inc.

Wingard, D. L., Suarez, L., & Barrett-Connor, E. (1983). The sex differential in mortality from all causes and ischemic heart disease. *American Journal of Epidemiology, 117,* 165–172.

Appendix
Dependent and Predictor
Variables

DEPENDENT VARIABLES:
INITIAL INTERVIEW

Health Status

Self-rated health status
No. of days not well due to illness or
    injury, past 2 weeks
No. of chronic health problems in
    past year
    No. of named chronic conditions
    No. of other frequent or repeated
    symptoms
    No. of impairments
Medically coded chronic problems
    (coded by Reason For Visit
    Classification; see Schneider,
    Appleton, and McLemore,
    1979):
No. of chronic diseases (D)
No. of chronic symptoms (S)
No. of injuries with chronic out-
    comes (J)
Chronic conditions in past year:
    Fatal conditions:
        Heart trouble (including high
        blood pressure)
        Heart trouble ever (past year or
        earlier)
        Respiratory or lung condition
        Diabetes or thyroid condition
        Stomach or intestinal condition
    Nonfatal conditions:
        Chronic skin condition
        Chronic musculoskeletal condi-
        tion
        Other allergies (excluding hay
        fever)
        Chronic eye or ear condition
        (excluding blindness, hearing
        loss)

Impairment due to old accident
    or injury
Female-dominant conditions:
    Other blood circulation con-
    ditions (including varicose
    veins and hemorrhoids; excl.
    heart disease, high blood
    pressure)
    Anemia or other blood system
    condition
    Nervous system condition
    (largely migraine)
Impairments:
    Impairment due to old accident
    or injury
    Congenital anomalies ("physic-
    al problem since birth")

Health Behavior

No. of restricted activity days due to
    illness or injury, past 2 weeks
No. of restricted activity days due to
    illness or injury, past year
    No. of days stayed in bed, past
    year
Job limitations due to health or
    physical problem
    (0=no limitation, 1=can work but
    limited in kind of job or amount
    of work at a job, 2=unable to
    have a paid job)
All limitations in social and physic-
    al function due to health
    (Index based on questions about
    job, housework/chores, free time
    activities, mobility/physical
    functioning, personal care)
No. of visits to medical doctor about
    own health in past year
    No. of visits for preventive care
    No. of visits for curative care
No. of drugs currently used for
    chronic problems

If any preventive drugs taken regularly

   No. of preventive drugs taken regularly (all R) (excl. contraceptives and other female products)

DEPENDENT VARIABLES: DAILY HEALTH RECORDS

NOTE: all items are for 6-week period.

Health Status

Daily physical feeling
   ("How did you feel physically today?"; 1=wonderful to 10=terrible; average for diary period)

No. of symptomatic days
   ("Did you have any symtoms or discomforts today?")

No. of health problems
   No. of "very serious" problems
   No. of "somewhat serious" problems
   No. of "not very serious" problems

Total no. of symptoms (Reason For Visit Classification's Symptom Module; see Schneider et al., 1979)
   No. of general symptoms
   No. of psychological/mental symptoms
   No. of nervous system symptoms (mostly headache)
   No. of cardiovascular/lymphatic system symptoms
   No. of eyes/ears symptoms
   No. of respiratory symptoms
   No. of digestive symptoms
   No. of genitourinary symptoms
   No. of skin/nails/hair symptoms
   No. of musculoskeletal symptoms

Causes of health problems (Reason For Visit Classification's Disease and Injuries/Adverse Effects Modules, and a new Other Cause Module developed for the study):
   No. of disease problems (D)
   No. of injuries/adverse effects problems (J)
   No. of problems due to other causes (K)

Health Behavior

No. of restricted activity days due to symptoms
   No. of days stayed in bed
   No. of days cut down on household chores or errands

No. of days with curative medical care for symptoms

No. of days with preventive medical care

No. of days talked with family or friends about symptoms (lay consultation)

No. of days took pills, medicine, or treatments for any reason ("drugs")

Total no. of drugs taken over diary period

Purposes of drugs:
   No. of curative drugs taken
   No. of drugs taken for asymptomatic chronic conditions
   No. of preventive drugs taken

Prescription status:
   No. of nonprescription drugs taken
   No. of prescription drugs taken

PREDICTORS

Lifestyle

Cigarett smoking (SMOKE)
   Currently smoke cigarettes, Don't smoke now but used to regularly, Don't smoke now and never did regularly (includes never smoked)

Alcohol consumption (DRINK)

Drank 15+ days in past month, Drank 1 to 14 days in past month, Didn't drink in past month but used to regularly (1+ days per month), Didn't drink in past month and never did regularly, Never had alcoholic beverage

Usual no. of hours of sleep per day (SLEEP)

Relative weight (RELWGT)

R's weight divided by midpoint of observed weight range for healthy U. S. adults (ages 18 to 74) of same height and sex, medium build assumed (see Frisancho, 1986: Tables 18, 24)

General level of physical activity each day (PHYSACTV)

1=none to 4=very much

Hours of strenuous leisure activity per week (STRENACTV)

0=none, 1=1 hour or less, 2=2-3, 3=4-5, 4=6-10, 5=more than 10

If any health hazards at job or home (HAZARDS)

Roles

Current employment status (EMPL)

0=nonemployed, 1=currently employed (working for pay)

Current marital status (MARR)

Currently married or "living together", Widowed, divorced, separated, Never married

Number of own preschool children in household (YOUNGCHD)

Feeling about main role (job or housework) (ROLEFEEL)

1=unqualified dislike to 5=unqualified like

Stress

General well being in past year (GB)

1=worst life you could expect to 10=best life you could expect

Recent stress (ACUTESTRESS)

Index based on 4 items about past month: nervousness, under strain or pressure, relaxed, anxious or upset

Persistent stress (CHRONICSTRESS)

Index based on 3 times about how often: work faster than like to get everything done, worry about future, have the chance to do things you like

Number of stressful life events in past year (LIFEEVENTS)

Socioeconomic

Educational attainment (EDUC)

Total family income for this year (INCOME)

Health Attitudes

NOTE: "HB" means the item is used as a predictor for health behavior only. Items in this section tap concepts in the Health Belief Model (Becker, 1974; Becker, Maiman, Kirscht, Haefner, & Drachman, 1977).

Value of health compared to other things in life (VALUE)

1=less than anything to 5=more than anything

Health responsibility (HLTHRESP)

Who cares for ill household members: 1=someone else, 2=everyone for self or whole family helps, 3=respondent

If respondent (R) would cut down usual activities for specific symptoms (IFCUTDOWN)

Index based on 8 symptoms; 1=not likely at all to 5=very likely; HB

If R would seek medical help for specific symptoms (IFSEEKCARE)

Index based on 6 symptoms; 1=take care of it yourself, 2=wait awhile and see doctor if it continues, 3=see doctor as soon as possible, 4=go to emergency room; HB

How much R thinks behaviors contribute to health (POSHEALTH)

Index based on 4 items about preventive medical care and lifestyle; 1=not at all to 5=a lot

If R thinks specific symptoms are signs of illness (SIGNS)

Index based on 8 symptoms; count of Yes

Vulnerability to illness, compared to age peers (VULNERABLE)

1=a lot less often to 5=a lot more often

Fatalism about causes of illness (HLC/CHANCE)

Index based on 2 Health Locus of Control items (Wallston, Wallston, & DeVellis, 1978): "Good health is largely a matter of good fortune" and "No matter what I do, if I am going to get sick I will".

If restricted activity helps R get better (EFFIC/RESTACT)

1=not at all to 5=a lot; HB

If following doctor's advice helps R get better (EFFIC/MDADV)

1=not true at all to 5=very true; HB

Psychological

Feelings of mastery in life (MASTERY)

Index based on 3 items about: feeling helpless with life problems, doing anything you set mind to, ability to change important things

Self-esteem (SELFESTEEM)

Index based on 3 items about: feeling useless, having good qualities, having more respect for self

Resistance to stress (POSITIVESIDE)

"I'm better off when I look only on the positive side of my life."

Structural/Enabling

NOTE: Andersen's model of health services access and use (Aday, Andersen, & Fleming, 1980; Andersen, 1968) guided the development of some items in this section.

How often R feels rushed (RUSHED)

"How much of the time do you feel rushed, that you don't have enough time to do the things you want or have to do?"; 1=never to 5=always

Number of committed hours per week (HOURS)

For job, commuting, household/ child care, volunteer work, and other regularly scheduled activities

How difficult it is to restrict activities when ill (DIFFIC/RESTACT)

1=not at all to 5=very; HB

Difficulty in leaving job

1=not at all to 5=very; HB

If R has health insurance (IFINSURED); HB

If R has a regular medical doctor or clinic (REGULAR); HB

How much R knows about health and disease, compared to age peers (KNOW)

1=much less to 5=much more; HB

Health Reporting Behavior

NOTE: all items rated by interviewer.

R's interest in the interview (INTEREST)
  1=not at all to 5=very

R's impatient to finish interview (IMPATIENCE)
  1=not at all to 5=very
R's ability to recall health actions in past year (RECALL)
  1=a lot to 5=not at all

11 Population Models of Gender Differences in Mortality, Morbidity, and Disability Risks

Kenneth G. Manton

This chapter addresses both substantive and methodological tasks in modeling population gender differences in morbidity, disability, and mortality. The first task is substantive and involves examining sex differences in the age trajectory of the linkages of morbidity, disability, and mortality in several types of data. The second task is methodological. It involves a review of population-based models of morbidity and mortality in order to show how biologically realistic population models of health changes at advanced ages can be developed, and how such biologically realistic population models can be used as tools to integrate scientific findings on the nature of sex differences in the aging process across a number of different levels of biological organization.

If biologically realistic models can be developed that are consistent with the different types of information available on aging changes at different levels of biological organization, then information from those different levels can be meaningfully integrated and contributions to the level of scientific knowledge at each level can be greatly enhanced. For example, a population model whose mathematical structure is designed to be consistent with clinical and laboratory findings about the age-related evolution of specific disease processes at the individual, organ, and cellular level can more realistically identify the sources of sex differences in aging processes and morbidity risks in population data than models without such features.

Research reported in this chapter was supported by HCFA cooperative agreement no. 18-C-98641, NIA grant no. AG-01159, NIA grant no. AG07025, and NIA grant no. AG07198.

Alternately, the application of a biologically motivated model to the analysis of population data can tell us if the observed patterns of population aging changes and morbidity and mortality risks are consistent with the implications of the biological principles used to construct the model. If the events and aging changes predicted from the model are not consistent with what is observed in the population, the discrepancy may result from the statistical implementation of the model or from deficiencies in the population data. It likewise could result from inadequacies in the biological theory and findings employed in the model's development. The success or failure in confirming basic biological findings at the population level is an important step in validating those findings. We shall, in examples presented below, illustrate this iterative process of model construction, empirical tests on population data, and the evaluation of the model's performance in terms of its biological implications for several dimensions of gender differences in aging, disability and mortality.

To accomplish these two tasks we present both substantive and methodological analyses. Several sources of data will be examined in our substantive analyses, including: (a) data on sex differences in disability and mortality linkages from the 1982 and 1984 National Long-Term Care Surveys; (b) conditions reported as causing disability for different age and sex groups from that survey; (c) sex specific models of select disease processes applied to mortality data from the national vital statistics system; and (d) results on sex differences using more detailed process models of human aging and mortality, applied to data from longitudinal community based studies. Methodologically, we will examine the differences between statistical hazard models and mathematical models of aging processes and show how biologically realistic models can be developed that integrate data from multiple sources.

HUMAN AGING AND MORTALITY: BASIC CONCEPTS

Several factors contributing to sex differences in the trajectory of morbidity and mortality were discussed during the September 1987 Conference on Gender and Longevity sponsored by the National Institute on Aging. One factor is that part of the sex differences is due to hormonal status; the hormonal status of premenopausal women apparently being protective against cardiovascular mortality—a finding consistent with sex differences in the distribution of lipoproteins (i.e., higher HDL levels in females). Postmenopausal shifts in hormonal status, in contrast, seem to be associated with a convergence of male/female circulatory disease risks at advanced ages and to the production of the acute and chronic sequelae of osteoporosis. Hormonal status also seems linked to the risk of various female (e.g., breast) and male (prostatic) cancer risks. A second factor is that women appear to have different and potentially stronger immune systems—a factor that, paradoxically, also leads to women having generally greater risk of autoimmune disorders like systemic lupus erythematosus and rheumatoid arthritis. A third factor, in contrast to the above two constitutional factors, is that sex-role differences in exposure to stress, alcohol, smoking, and work-place hazards leads to higher male risks for a number of chronic respiratory and circulatory problems.

The problem is to develop models for analyzing population level data that can consistently represent individual variation in such biomedical and epidemiological factors. Unfortunately, standard strategies for analyzing *population* health data may not provide results consistent with the underlying biological mechanisms. It is possible, however, with the appropriate concepts to develop population models that do permit such analyses.

Specification of Standard Hazard Models

As a first step in developing satisfactory population models we should first consider what the standard hazard analyses used by most social scientists and demographers imply about the mortality and aging at the individual level. Consider, for example, Figure 11.1.

In this figure there are three lines. Line A represents the "observed" hazard function that describes the increase in the risk of the event as a function of age. Line B represents the hazard function when the variation in risk due to some significant covariates are statistically controlled. We can see that the hazard function estimated with covariates tends to rise more sharply as a function of age. This is because such hazard functions actually represent an "age residual"—or the uncertainty of the time of death for an individual. Thus, when covariates are added, uncertainty about the individuals's age at death is reduced and the hazard function must rise more rapidly to reflect the reduced uncertainty or error variability of the age at death. The limit of this process is illustrated by line C which shows that, when all covariates necessary to exactly predict the time of death of an individual are in the model, the hazard function collapses to a spike at the precise age at death.

Thus, Figure 11.1 shows that the concept of an age variable "hazard"

Figure 11.1 The effect of covariates on population hazard function.

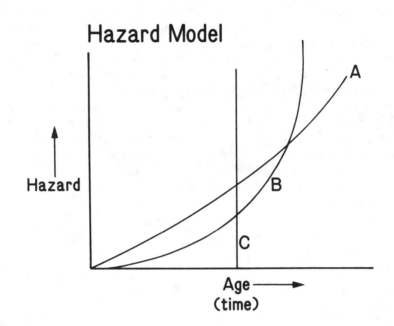

is meaningful only in aggregate or population terms. At the individual level the hazard model describes aging processes as a simple discrete change where a person can only be in one of two states, that is the "alive" state or the "dead" state. In this case the age-specific hazard rate adopts only the values 0 or 1.0. Such a model does not describe features of age-related changes in biological state. Covariates are only used to statistically "stratify" the population. The coefficients for covariates in the hazard function do *not* describe parameters of the aging process.

Specification of Two-Component Model

In contrast to the hazard model described above are models of human aging and mortality that directly describe the individual aging process. To do this a model must describe the interaction of at least *two* component processes. One component process is necessary to describe changes in physiological status with age. The second component pro-

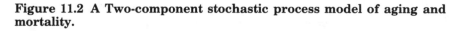

Figure 11.2 A Two-component stochastic process model of aging and mortality.

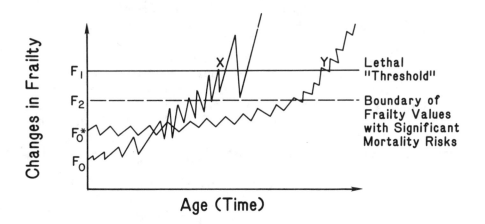

cess is necessary to describe the "threshold" beyond which the physiology of the organism is inadequate to sustain life. Such a model is illustrated in Figure 11.2

In Figure 11.2 we do *not* plot the hazard rate as a function of age, but changes in the physiological status of a person as a function of age. In this figure we have, for simplicity, represented physiological status by a single dimension labelled "frailty", which is directly related to his/her homeostatic capacity (i.e., his/her ability to resist death). In all practical applications we will generalize the model to represent changes in a multidimensional physiological space.

A person's change in frailty is represented by curved, jagged lines. The curves beginning at F_0 and F_0^* represent persons whose genetically determined initial frailty is F_0 and F_0^*. The increases in "frailty" with time/age can either be a function of intrinsic differences in the rate of physiological aging or the accumulated effect of different environmental exposures. For the current discussion let us assume that both persons are exposed to the same environment so that differences in the long-term change of the curves with time/age is a result of intrinsic aging processes. The jagged lines represent the interaction of (a) short-term changes in frailty due to environmental "shocks" and (b) the individual's ability to maintain homeostasis in the face of those environmental shocks. The fact that there is greater variance in the trajectory of frailty at advanced ages for F_0 is due to an assumed weakening of homeostatic forces at advanced ages. The solid line at frailty level F_1 represents a "lethal threshold." An infant whose frailty value due to intrinsic endowment is above F_1 will be "still born." When the trajectory of frailty for a person first exceeds the line F_1, "death" occurs. This occurs at age X for the person starting at F_0 and at age Y for the person beginning at frailty F_0^*. In the discussion below, the lethal "threshold" will be replaced by a lethal "region" (e.g., points above the dotted line at F_2) with the probability of death increasing as one proceeds to higher levels of frailty. Furthermore, the frailty trajectory for the person beginning at F_0^*, though initially higher than F_0, increases less rapidly with age and thus represents a "slower" aging process. Note that the two curves are not proportional to one another and, at certain points, F_0 is stochastically at a lower level of frailty. Aging represented by this type of two component process model can be far more general than for models based on simple Gompertz or Weibull functions.

Biologists are well aware of the need for a two component model to describe individual aging changes and mortality. Several examples of such models are presented in Strehler (1977). Unfortunately, there has been little work on developing statistical strategies to apply such models to human population data. Generally, such models are reduced to unidimensional form before application to data. Even the model in Sacher and Trucco (1962) was reduced to the unidimensional case when evaluated empirically. Specifically, Sacher and Trucco (1962) showed that, when one root to the solution of the differential equation describing physiological aging changes dominates, the solution can be approximated by a Gompertz function. The empirical application of this model then typically involved assessing the fit of a Gompertz function to human mortality data (e.g., Sacher, 1977). The Gompertz coefficients estimated from human mortality data are then interpreted in terms of their implications for theory and empirical observations made in other types of studies. For example, the Gompertz parameter estimates implies a specific rate of loss of a physiological function, which then can be compared to the rate observed in a longitudinally followed population or observations made on the basis of laboratory studies. However, even in those evaluations not all the available data is typically exploited. For example, the Sacher–Trucco model is based on the assumption that age changes in functions were linear—there is no simple continuous function that describes the individual trajectories of functional loss.

The Need for a Multidimensional Population Model

The problems with this approach to the empirical application of the two component models are twofold. First, the assumption that the process can be reduced to a single dimension at advanced ages is questionable. Neither the change in physiological state, nor the nature of the mode of failure of the organism, is likely to be unidimensional. That is, the human organism is a complex biological entity composed of multiple, interacting organ systems each with its own age trajectory of loss of function. The argument that the organism, at an advanced age, falls into a type of temporal "lock-step" in terms of loss of physiological capacity is a rather grand assumption that requires investigation. One could observe rapid loss of homeostasis due to the interdepencence of organ systems without having the aging changes in the cells of each organ being directly affected by aging processes in other organ systems.

Second, it is likely that the "modes of failure" of the organism are multiple and possibly interact. We use the term "modes of failure" as a more general term than "cause of death" because while the term cause of death refers to the (possibly multiple) pathological conditions initiating the physiological processes resulting in death, the term mode of failure represents the set of significant pathological milestones emerging over time in the processes leading to death. Thus, the cause of death model requires defining the point in time at which the failure process initiated (a necessarily somewhat arbitrary point), while the mode of failure concept does not. An example of a mode of failure analysis conducted by taking the death certificate report of medical conditions at the time of death as "fixed" is given in Manton, Stallard, and Poss (1980). An alternative mode of failure analysis that views patterns of manifested conditions as stochastic is the multivariate Grade of Membership analysis of data from the Yale EPESE study reported by Berkman, Manton, and Singer (1989). Thus, the lethal "region" identified in Figure 11.2 may actually be multiple regions with different properties and boundaries for each "mode" of failure.

These arguments suggest that population models must be multivariate and deal with multiple, possibly interdependent modes of failure, in order to be biologically realistic. Such multivariate, multiple outcome models will provide the necessary tools for biologists to construct (and validate) their models of human aging and mortality. Arguments about whether the Gompertz or the Weibull function better describe aging dynamics are based on the strong assumption that the aging process is unidimensional and does not directly allow the detail on the operation of the aging process in current theoretical systems to be directly evaluated (e.g., Economos, 1982).

BIOLOGICALLY MOTIVATED MODELS OF SEX DIFFERENCES IN HUMAN AGING AND MORTALITY

In developing practical, biologically motivated models to analyze sex differences in aging processes and mortality we must also deal with the observational plan under which the available data were generated (for example, different types of population data will be rich on one type of data dimension and poor on another). National cause specific mortality data are available at the individual level for a number of years and represent all deaths occurring in the U.S. in each year—permitting the identification and analysis of rare events, the recording of deaths at the most extreme ages, and the examination of geographic differences in cause specific mortality trends as well as cohort differences. Few other data sets have the necessary scope and volume of data necessary to analyze such factors. Such data are, unfortunately, weak in terms of the measurement of physiological covariates. As a consequence, models developed to analyze this type of demographic data depend heavily on ancillary biological data and theory to construct a detailed internal structure for the model. The amount of detail in the model that can be *directly* estimated is limited.

In contrast there are longitudinal studies of select community populations for which detailed, repeated physiological measurements are made. From this type of data the parameters of a very detailed process model can be estimated directly. Unfortunately such data usually (a) do not contain adequate numbers of deaths at the most advanced ages, (b) do not contain adequate numbers of cases to identify detailed differences between cohorts, (c) do not represent geographic differences in mortality and morbidity differences and (d) do not have adequate numbers of rare morbid and lethal events.

To deal with the characteristics of the different types of data one needs different types of analytic models. Below we will discuss two basic types of models—one a discrete state, continuous time stochastic process and the second a multivariate continuous state, continuous time model. We will show how the continuous state model can be viewed as the natural generalization of the discrete state model for large numbers of states (Manton, 1988a) and then discuss how each can be used to evaluate sex differences in aging processes and mortality.

Discrete State-Continuous Time Aging Models

In the previous section we discussed how the standard hazard models used in social science data did not describe the population variation of aging processes and outcomes in biologically meaningful ways. Such hazard models have been typically used in demographic analyses when describing discrete changes like death. The question is, "are there models of discrete changes that are biologically meaningful and which can be used to describe the type of two component process represented in Figure 11.2 and which can be estimated from demographic data?" The answer is yes, that the class of models described as stochastic compartment models (Jaquez, 1972) are discrete state, continuous time-process models that can be applied to the analysis of complex processes in which certain stages in the process (i.e., physiological state changes) are only partially observed. The original application of these models was in pharmacokinetics where the rate of ingestion and excretion of a drug (and its metabolites) could be observed but *not* the intermediate metabolic stages. These could be inferred by developing models of those intermediate metabolic stages using ancillary biological theory and linking them by the appropriate mathematical forms to the input and output compartments (e.g., Matis & Wehrly, 1979). Similarly the flow of a population from birth, through various health states to death, can be viewed as a type of population "metobolism." Thus, the extension of these compartment modeling techniques to population analyses is based on certain natural analogies between the two types of phenomena.

Case Example: Lung Cancer

To illustrate, let us examine lung cancer mortality. In Figure 11.3 a model is presented composed of physiological states and transitions which, with appropriate ancillary biological theory and data, is estimable from population and cause specific mortality counts (Manton & Stallard, 1982).

In this figure we see that persons can live in one of three health states (i.e., well, latent tumor growth, and tumor treatment). These three states can be viewed as describing the changes in frailty level in Figure 11.2 with two simple models of failure, that is two types of lethal regions.

Actually the age trajectory of state changes is far more complex than simply being in one of the three health states so that, in order to estimate the transition rates, one must make them time dependent functions of continuous biological changes in each of those states. For example, to estimate λ_1 (i.e., the incidence of a tumor), we must posit a function describing the age-specific risk of a cell losing growth control. In the case of lung cancer (and many other solid tumors; Cook, Felling-

Figure 11.3 Compartments and transitions of a stochastic process model of lung cancer.

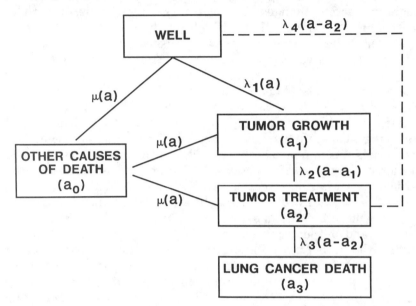

ham, & Doll, 1969) the dynamics can be related to what has been called the "multihit" or "multistage" model of carcinogenesis (Armitage & Doll, 1954, 1961). This is a model of the events that occur in the cell nucleus that lead to loss of cellular growth control and the growth of a tumor from a single cell origin. In effect, this model assumes that growth control is lost after a series of "m" nonlethal changes in the cell nucleus. This type of cellular failure process leads to the following Weibull function for the age specific risk ($\lambda_1(a)$) of the initiation of the tumor in an individual:

$$\lambda_1(a) = \alpha \, a^{m-1} \tag{1}$$

This function describes the age increase in the risk of the onset of malignant tumor growth from a single cell as a function of age raised to the m-1st power. The factor α reflects both the product of the probabilities of each of the m changes in the cell nucleus and the number of cells in the organ system of interest. If the order of the cell changes is not important to the likelihood of a tumor starting we have the "multi-hit" model as in equation (1) above. If the changes are necessarily sequenced then the term α in (1) would include a combinatorial factor indicating that only one sequence of cell changes will produce a tumor. On biological grounds, though the value of α estimated from population data is the same for the multi-hit and stage models, the different models have very different implications for the probability that one of the m errors has occurred, that is in the multi-stage models the probability of a cell error must be much higher because certain sequences of changes will not produce a malignant tumor. To discriminate between the two theoretical scenarios direct data on cellular changes is required, that is from the population analyses only certain classes of theoretical statements can be evaluated.

Features of the Model at the Individual Level

The multistage/hit model of tumor kinetics has several important biological implications that can be evaluated in laboratory studies. One feature is that the model assumes that each of the cell errors has a probability of occurrence that is independent of age—an observation that has been made in several animal studies (Peto et al., 1975). Other evidence would suggest that the error rate might increase with age, although an acceleration of the age rate of tumor incidence at very advanced ages is not generally observed. This may be due, as discussed below, to the dependence of tumor expression on other biological functions that change with age. A second implication of the model is that dose-response functions will be of a specific power form. Specifically, if an exposure promotes *one* type of error the above model would suggest a linear dose response function. If the probability of two types of errors are affected by a given exposure, then the dose-response function will be quadratic. Such power law formulations of dose-response have been found to be applicable for a wide variety of exposures (Whittemore, 1977). A third type of evidence relates to laboratory and clinical studies. One set of studies involves verification that certain viruses or chemical exposures cause discrete changes in the DNA in the cell nucleus or the "turning on" of certain oncogenes and that these events are associated with loss of growth control. A related type of evidence is that certain tumor types, when occurring in families with a history of a specific disease, have an age increase with a power of m one less than in families without such a history—suggesting the existence of a discrete genetic defect predisposing to the disease (e.g., Knudson, Strong, & Anderson, 1973). A related type of evidence is that, for certain types of tumors, the value of m is smaller in families with a history of other disease than for families without a history. For example, in certain childhood tumors, the value of m is two in families without a history, and one when a history is present. The smaller value suggests that the familial predisposition is a result of one of the $m=2$ genetic errors necessary for the disease to occur to be present in genetic code of the families with a past disease history (Knudson, Strong, & Anderson, 1973). The recent identification of specific oncogenes that are apparently continuously producing growth factors by being stuck in the "on" position in malignant tumors (e.g., the HER-2 oncogene for breast cancer) also suggest a type of discrete change underlying the initiation of tumor growth.

In sum, there is considerable biological evidence supporting the reasonableness of the mathematical form of equation (1) as a model of the age dependence of the risk of tumor initiation. It is applicable even if certain cell errors are "reversible" (e.g., Watson, 1977). Thus biological evidence and theory have been used to specify an indivudual level model of changes in the cell nucleus associated with the risk of disease onset. This model is logically equivalent to the linear dynamic equations of our two component model, that is, it describes a time-directed change in the physiological state of the individual (i.e., the "state" of the organ as described by the average number of cells in the target organ that have "one" error, the number with "two" errors, etc.). The problem is how to relate this individual level model to the expression of age-related disease and mortality at the population level. This involves models of: (a) the distribution of individual level processes in the population, and (b) the lethal threshold that identifies the probability of death given that the physiological changes indicated by equation (1) have reached a given level.

Modeling at the Population Level

To introduce the first component in the model the features of the model likely to vary over individuals have to be identified. For lung cancer this is most likely to be the probability of each of the m errors whose product are reflected in α. A general model of the distribution of individual values of α (say α_i) is the gamma distribution which, when combined with the individual level model in (1), yields as the population model for the risk of tumor onset (Manton & Stallard, 1979),

$$\bar{\lambda}_1(a) = \alpha\, a^{m-1}/[1 + \alpha\, a^m/(ms)] \qquad (2)$$

where the age rate of increase in the risk of tumor onset in the population (where $\bar{\lambda}_1(a)$ represents the average risk among survivors to age a) is slowed below that predicted by the Weibull by the factor in the divisor that is a function of the gamma shape parameter, s. Large values of s (i.e., greater than 0.5) are interpretable as describing the distribution of risk factors for the disease in the population (i.e., the relation of the shape parameter to the number of dimensions n affecting survival is $n = 2s$; Manton & Stallard, 1981). Small values of s (i.e., less than 0.1) are interpretable as measures of the proportion of the population most susceptible to the risk of tumor onset (Manton &

Stallard, 1982). The "slowing" of the age rate of increase in the population is thus due to death first occurring to individuals with the highest α values.

The second model component involves introducing the lethal "threshold." For the multistage/hit tumor kinetics this is a function of the rate of growth of the tumor with the risk of death being proportional to tumor size. Clinical studies give us evidence on the amount of time for the tumor to double in size with 30 to 40 doublings typically required before the tumor is of lethal mass (Archambeau, Heller, Akanuma, & Lubell, 1970). This can be introduced by replacing "a" in equation (1) with "a − t," where t is the time for the tumor to reach a lethal size. The modeling problem is to define a biologically meaningful model for λ_2 to estimate t. In the lung cancer case we assumed that the tumor grew exponentially or, $\lambda_2 (a - a_1) = k_0 \exp[B(a - a_1)]$ (where $t = a - a_1$) and that the exponent governing the rate of growth (i.e., B) is log-normally distributed over individuals. The model can also be generalized to represent additional discrete changes in health state, for example, the change from unobserved to observed "treated" tumor growth state by redefining t as equal to $a_1 - a_2$. Functions then have to be defined to model the component transitions separately. This could be done in the current example by using data on clinical survival from the National Cancer Institute (NCI) SEER data by isolating from the total time from the initiation of tumor growth to death, separate times for either death or "cure" to occur. In Figure 11.3, $\lambda_3(a - a_2)$ can be viewed as the case fatality rate based on our model of tumor growth and the transition rate, $\lambda_4(a - a_2)$ represents the cure rate. Estimation of transitions and state descriptive parameters for the model in Figure 11.3 for the national population requires utilization of insights and evidence from (a) biological models of carcinogenesis and tumor kinetics, (b) data from clinical and epidemiological studies of individual differences in the risks of tumor onset and the rate of tumor growth, and (c) data from multiple vital statistics, epidemiological, and clinical sources on cancer mortality and survival.

Adjustment for Competing Risk

In addition to the functions describing the disease process, one also needs to introduce the adjustment for competing risks by including the effect of other forces of mortality—the μ terms. If the three μ terms in Figure 11.3 are different (i.e., the risk of death from "other causes" for persons with a lung tumor growing is higher than for persons without a lung tumor because persons with lung tumors have higher than average tobacco consumption rates), then we can represent a dependent competing risk effect in the model, that is an interaction of physiological state with multiple modes of failure. This can be done with ancillary data on risk factor exposure effects on other major causes of death.

By combining the complex functions for tumor onset, tumor growth, and clinical data on survival (see methods in Manton & Stallard, 1982) one can estimate the distribution of persons in each of the three states and the distribution of persons at different levels of the process operating in each state. For example, in Figure 11.4 we present the distribution of time spent in the tumor growth state which is a direct function of (a) tumor growth kinetics, (b) the risk of a tumor passing the observable threshold, and (c) the risk of dying first of some other cause of death.

Application of the Model

Previously we discussed how biological theory could be used in the construction of a model of the individual dynamics of tumor growth which, when combined across persons, defined a site-specific cancer mortality model at the population level. In analyses of population and mortality data, where the amount of information on the biological state of each individual is limited, there is a heavy dependence on modeling strategies that use ancillary biological theory and data.

Having constructed such a model it can be applied to the extensive national population and mortality data available. Such an analysis has three advantages. First, it provides estimates of the parameters of the process at the national level. That is, though the biological theory may dictate the functional form of components of the model, the numerical values of the parameters in the national population may be quite different than in highly select clinical populations and in vitro studies from which the form of specific components of the model are derived. Second, the population data allows assessment of the variation of parameters across a number of population subgroups of importance in addition to sex. For example, the differential exposures of various male and female birth cohorts may alter their rate parameters. National data are rich enough to estimate rate parameters for different cohorts. Other subgroups of interest may involve geographic differences, urban–rural differences, and occupational exposures. A third important use of these models is to validate the biological theory used in their construction. That is, the population models generate predictions of sex, cohort, and age-specific mortality rates. These predictions may or may not be close to the observed population values. If the predictions are not close to the observed values this raises the possibility of deficiencies in the biological theory used to construct the model. Thus, population analyses with biologically motivated models

Figure 11.4 Hypothetical distribution of tumor growth latency times based on parameters derived from model of U.S. white male lung cancer mortality.

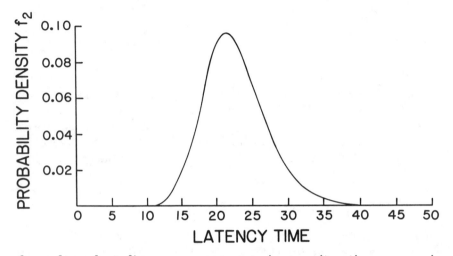

of age-dependent disease processes requires an iterative process in which biological theory and evidence are used to construct a model; those models are applied to data with the resulting ability to reproduce those data offering insights into the validity of the original biological theory and data.

Continuous State–Continuous Time Models

The compartment model described above represents the effects of aging-related physiological changes and, because there is continuous biological variation of persons within the three discrete states, the multidimensional analogue of the frailty distribution in this model has a combination of continuous and discrete components. However, building such a model using a wide range of ancillary data is a complex task. Furthermore, because parameters are indirectly estimated, the model requires large amounts of data. If such a model is not constructed, however, there is a significant likelihood that inferences about aging and morbidity processes from population data will be, at best, biologically naive and, at worst, incorrect. In certain studies, where the number of discrete states in one's model is large, problems arise because the data requirements become extreme. When the number of states is large it is necessary to use a generalization of the discrete state model (Gillespie, 1983). As the number of states increase they form a multivariate continuous state where changes in the distribution of the population are governed by stochastic differential equations. These equations result from "random" walk probabilistic equations in which the variation on state variables is continuous (Woodbury & Manton, 1977).

Monitoring Changes in Physiological States Over Time

Random walk models can be estimated from longitudinal studies of populations in which a number of physiological parameters are monitored over time (Manton & Woodbury, 1985). In this type of study we have the necessary data to directly estimate both types of process parameters described in Figure 11.2. Specifically, from survivors to a given time, we can model changes in physiological status by the simple autoregressive function,

$$x_{it+1} = u_0 + C \cdot Age + A\, x_{it} + e_{it+1} \tag{3}$$

This simple equation says that the value of a given measured physiological variable j at a time $t + 1$ can be predicted from: a constant (u_0); a term representing systematic changes with age (time) (C); a set of regression coefficients representing the dependency of j on itself and on all $J - 1$ other covariates measured at the prior time (t); and stochastic disturbances (e_{it+1}).

This simple linear equation can describe two interesting features of the physiological dynamics of aging.

Tracking

Tracking represents the "persistence" of an individual's physiological state with, potentially, age trends, period effects, and linear dependencies on other physiological variables super-imposed. Tracking might be represented by making one of the parameters in (3) individual specific, for example,

$$x_{it+1} = u_{0(i)} + C \cdot Age + A \cdot x_{it} + e_{it+1}, \tag{4}$$

so that there is an individual constant underlying the age rate of change of each of the j factors. If "tracking" is included in a model, this naturally has significant effects on the estimates of the magnitude of stochastic effect or shocks (i.e., the size of e_{it+1}) because a larger component of the variation of physiological characteristics is attributed to fixed individual effects.

In representing sex differences in the physiological dynamics described in (4) we could hypothesize several different types of effects. There could simply be a mean shift [i.e., one additional term for sex in equation (1), say u_{0F} for females and u_{0M} for males, e.g., Woodbury & Manton, 1983], different age trends (i.e., C is different for males and females), or different physiological dynamics (i.e., matrix A is different for males and females).

Homeostasis

The second type of dynamic effect is homeostasis. This can be represented by the equation

$$x_h = (I-A)^{-1} u_0 \tag{5}$$

When combined with force of regression this represents the set of risk-factor values toward which the physiological dynamics tends to drive an individual's physiological state. The force of regression can be written as

$$-u_{it} = (I-A) (x_{it} - x_h) \tag{6}$$

where u_{it} is the rate of change of physiological values predicted by the regression function. This change vector is a function of (a) the distance between the homeostatic point (x_h) and the person's current set of physiological values (x_{it}), and (b) the regression matrix A. Again, if the regression dynamics are different for males and females the homeostatic point and the regression effect will also be different. It is also possible that sex differences in homeostasis will vary with age (e.g., if A is made age dependent). Naturally, if dynamic equation (3) or (4) is different for males and females, then the homeostatic point will be different for males and females.

Modeling the Risk of Death

A second component of the process describes the probability that a person at a specific point in the physiological space will die. This component can be written as

$$\mu(x_{it}) = (\alpha e^{\theta t}) (\mu_0 + b^T x_{it} + \tfrac{1}{2} x_{it} B x_{it}^T B x_{it}) \tag{7}$$

which says that the risk of death (μ) for persons with physiological characteristics, x_{it}, is a quadratic function of those values times an age dependent function ($\alpha e^{\theta t}$) like the Gompertz, where, for simplicity, we assume that t indexes both age and time. Equation (7) represents a multivariate generalization of Gompertzian aging dynamics to the case that those dynamics are made functions of *both* (a) fixed environmental and genetic factors (i.e., the Gompertz function is effectively made specific to the profile of physiological values that a person exhibits at a given point in time), and (b) to the dynamics of those physiological variables (i.e., equation (4); the model describing temporal changes in the profile of physiological values for an individual). Thus, a Gompertzian (or Weibull) model of intrinsic aging changes can be extended to include a detailed model of changes in physiological state. Furthermore, if we made the hazard, μ, specific to different "modes of failure," the model can represent multiple outcomes as well as being multivariate. Furthermore, since the μ for different modes of failure are dependent on a common set of physiological variables for the individual a natural type of interaction or competition between those modes of failure is represented in the model.

As for the dynamic equations, different terms in equation (7) can be made sex specific. For example, the effects of risk factors on mortality can be quite different for males and females meaning that the coefficients in b and B may be different. Alternately, the Gompertz function describing age-related change in mortality, net of the effect of the covariates, could have different coefficients implying different intrinsic age rates of change in the probability of being in a lethal region for males and females.

Modeling at the Population Level

Equations (4) and (7) describe the risk of death and physiological change for an individual. As such we could select any functional form for these equations. If, however, we wish to examine the aggregate changes in a population, we must mathematically study the interaction of the dynamics and mortality to determine how population parameters will change. Mathematical analyses show that, for the mathematical forms described above, the difference equations (8)–(12) below, describe how the characteristics of the population change (Woodbury & Manton, 1983).

For example, equation (8) shows that the probability of surviving to age $t + 1$ is a product of surviving to time t (S_t) and terms involving the means (ν) and variances (V) of the distributions of the J physiological parameters and terms (μ, b, and B) from the quadratic mortality functions,

$$S_{t+1} = S_t \left| I + V_j B_j \right|^{-1/2} \exp \left\{ \frac{\mu(\nu_t) + \mu(\nu_t^*)}{2} - 2\mu \left[\frac{\nu_t + \nu_2^*}{2} \right] \right\} \qquad (8)$$

The term S_t can be viewed as the probability of surviving to age t from a standard life table—except, of course, that equation (8) also implicitly contains our model of multivariate physiological change in that the parameters V and ν will change according to equation (4). The next two equations show how the mean and variance of the population distribution of physiological variables is altered by mortality, that is the mean (ν) and variance (V) is calculated for those people who are projected to survive to $t + 1$—hence the equations again contain coefficients from the quadratic hazard function.

$$V_t^* = (I + V_t B)^{-1} V_t \tag{9}$$

$$\nu_t^* = \nu_t - V_t^*(b + B \nu_t) \tag{10}$$

Finally, for those persons who survive to $t + 1$ we must change their physiological status by applying both the forces of deterministic (i.e., u and A) and stochastic (i.e., Σ_t) age dynamics

$$\nu_{t+1} = u_t + A \nu_t^* \tag{11}$$

$$V_{t+1} = \Sigma_t + A V_t^* A^T. \tag{12}$$

These five equations show how the dynamics of the aging and mortality selection processes for individuals interact over time to determine population changes. Other mathematical forms may not produce difference equations like (8)–(12) so that the relation of individual dynamics and mortality in those models may not be consistently related with population dynamics and mortality. Sex differences may be represented in either the dynamic or mortality equations and could suggest very different patterns of age change in (8)–(12). Such differences will be represented in the example presented below by different types of life-table functions. With such equations it is also possible to see how clinical and laboratory findings may be directly introduced into the modeling of the population. For example, if one knows that there is a specific mechanism determining the age rate of loss of renal function, that functional form could be introduced in C in (4) in the appropriate equations and estimated conditionally on other observed factors in the population.

SELECTED STUDIES OF SEX DIFFERENCES IN AGE-DEPENDENT MORBIDITY AND MORTALITY PROCESSES

In this section we illustrate the models described above. These examples are meant to show concretely the iterative process of interaction between population modeling and biological and clinical studies and *not* to be exhaustive review of gender differences in aging and mortality. The examples are presented in order of model sophistication. First, there is basic data on sex differences in individual transitions between morbidity, disability, and mortality. Second, we examine sex differences in the parameters of the tumor kinetics model estimated from population mortality data for several types of cancer (i.e., lung, breast, stomach). Finally, we examine sex differences in models of human aging and mortality estimated from longitudinal data on individuals from community epidemiological studies.

Sex Specific Patterns of Morbidity, Disability and Mortality

Below we present estimates for simple discrete state, discrete time models of health status change in the elderly population. These models are estimated from two national surveys: the 1982 and 1984 National Long-Term Care Survey (NLTCS).

A Discrete Time–Discrete State Model of Disability

The 1982–1984 NLTCS has two useful properties. Individuals interviewed in 1982 are reinterviewed in 1984 so that the health changes of persons can be followed. Secondly, a two-stage sampling procedure was used to increase the number of disabled persons that could be interviewed. As a consequence we have excellent precision for the health transitions of chronically disabled persons—a subpopulation of particular interest. From the surveys we can estimate the two-year risks of morbidity, disability, institutionalization, and mortality for the entire U.S. male and female population aged 65 and over in 1982. Estimates of these transitions, separately for males and females, are presented in Table 11.1

In the table the status of the population aged 65 and over in 1982 is presented down the left hand margin with the status of the population in 1984 presented across the top. The entries in the table represent the probability of a person in a given state in 1982 being in a given state in 1984. For example, for males who were not disabled in 1982, there was an 81.07% chance they would not be disabled in 1984, a 0.94% chance they would have 5 to 6 Activities of Daily Living (ADL) impaired in 1984, a 1.01% chance of being institutionalized in 1984 and a 10.72% chance of dying by 1984. In addition to dividing the population into nondisabled, institutional, and disabled community resident groups in 1982, the disabled community resident group is further divided into four subpopulations based on his/her level of disability (e.g., defined in terms of ADL and Instrumental Activities of Daily Living (IADL)). In

Table 11.1 The Two-Year (1982 to 1984) Probabilities of Changes in Disability, Institutional and Vital Stastus for Males (M) and Females (F) from the 1982 and 1984 National Long Term Care Survey

Functional, institutional and vital status in 1982	Not Disabled		IADL Disability		1-2 ADL Disabilities		3-4 ADL Disabilities		5-6 ADL Disabilities		Institutionalized		Deceased	
	M	F	M	F	M	F	M	F	M	F	M	F	M	F
Not Disabled	81.07	82.01	3.25	4.58	2.29	3.46	0.82	1.12	0.84	0.87	1.01	1.75	10.72	6.20
IADL Only	11.71	7.89	42.37	39.97	13.40	23.90	3.73	5.67	5.64	3.37	4.04	6.41	19.12	12.79
1-2 ADL	2.50	4.17	12.58	15.60	28.76	37.20	12.33	12.78	8.74	5.39	6.00	8.05	29.08	16.78
3-4 ADL	3.18	1.17	3.93	4.19	13.25	20.03	18.94	24.89	18.13	20.61	6.96	11.08	35.62	18.04
5-6 ADL	1.12	0.53	4.74	4.87	7.18	8.14	9.12	8.78	29.11	32.16	6.52	11.18	42.21	34.33
Persons reporting being institutionalized as of 4/1/82	0.73	0.47	0.90	0.70	0.99	0.40	0.89	0.97	0.74	0.93	48.06	58.71	47.68	37.82
Persons who started but did not complete household survey	4.69	5.57	7.64	7.75	5.71	11.66	4.94	8.21	5.53	9.52	7.26	18.90	64.24	38.38
Persons reporting being institutionalized after 4/1/82 but before the date of the screening interview	2.57	3.93	1.28	3.84	3.19	3.74	3.63	1.79	2.02	2.58	35.10	44.94	52.21	39.19

addition two groups are identified who report being institutionalized in 1982—these persons were identified, but not interviewed in 1982 (institutionalized persons *were* interviewed in 1984).

Several observations can be made about the table. First, the two-year mortality risks vary considerably across disability level. There is about a 4–(males) to 5½ (females) fold greater chance of death for persons with 5 to 6 ADL limitations in 1982 than for unimpaired persons in 1982. Second, there is a considerable chance of improving functional status over the two-year period—even for those with 5 to 6 ADL limitations (i.e., a total of 22.2% of those with 5 to 6 ADL limitations in 1982 have a lower level of impairment in 1984). Interestingly, persons with 3 to 4 ADL limitations have the lowest probability of remaining at the same impairment level—lower than for persons with 5 to 6 ADL impairments despite that group's higher mortality rates.

The transitions for persons who reported being in institutions on April 1, 1982 appears reasonable for long-term residents of nursing homes. Persons institutionalized after April 1, 1982, but before the screening interview (a lag of about 2 months), have both the highest risks of death (except for persons who started but did not complete the interview) *and* a high likelihood of improving function between 1982 and 1984.

Sex Differences in Disability and Mortality Transitions

The sex differences in the disability and mortality transitions are of greatest interest in Table 11.1. The likelihood of remaining nonimpaired over two years is similar for males (81.1%) and females (82.0%). This differs from prevalance estimates of disability in which females have a higher prevalence. The explanation of the difference between the incidence and prevalence rates are found in the sex-specific mortality rates at each level of impairment. At each level of impairment (and age), female mortality rates are significantly lower than for males. Thus, at each level of impairment females live longer than males so that the prevalence of females with disability is greater.

In a second analysis we stratified the two-year disability transitions for males and females by age. In the age-specific analyses we found confirmation that mortality rates for females were not only lower at every level of impairment but that the relation held at every age (Manton, 1988b).

To understand the greater survival of females at each disability level (and age) we examined the medical conditions reported by males and females as causing their disability (Table 11.2).

There are significant differences in the conditions reported as causing disability for males and females (Manton, 1988b). Ischemic heart disease, respiratory disease, and cancer are more prevalent among males than females. Interestingly, conditions that are viewed as risk factors for cardiovascular disease (e.g., diabetes mellitus, hypertension) are more prevalent among *females* suggesting a greater ability to tolerate exposure to these conditions without manifesting significant circulatory events. Indeed, despite the higher prevalence of diabetes and hypertension severe enough to cause chronic disability, even more diffuse circulatory damage (i.e., "other" circulatory diseases that include diffuse atherosclerotic disease), is more common for males. It may be that the premenopausal hormonal protective effects are strong enough to prevent or delay catastrophic circulatory degeneration—even in the face of diabetes and hypertension.

Females have higher risks of arthritis (including rheumatoid forms) than males (despite males' greater occupational risks)—indicative of females' greater tendency towards immunological disorders. Females also have higher reported risks of senile dementia than males for whom certain neurological disorders like Parkinson's are more often reported. In general, medical conditions that are viewed as more highly lethal (e.g., cancer, heart disease) are more frequently reported as causes of disability for males. Thus, there is evidence that the higher prevalence of disability among females is due to longer survival associated with sex differences in the pattern of causes of disability.

Models of Carcinogenesis in Males and Females

The sex differences in health and functional status changes were previously described with a simple discrete state, discrete time model. In this section examples are presented of population analyses using biologically motivated discrete state, continuous time process models. These analyses, because of limitations on the biological detail in the population data, rely heavily on ancillary biological data and theory.

Case Example: Breast Cancer

The first example is that of female breast cancer in the U.S. Though a number of etiological factors have been identified for breast cancer (e.g., MacMahon, Cole, & Brown, 1973), none of these has successfully explained the observation of the "Clemmsen's hook" (DeWaard, Baanders-VanHalewijn, & Huizinga, 1964), a slowing of the age rate of increase in mortality risks for a period about the age of menopause in occidental populations. This has stimulated a number of theories about the mechanisms of breast cancer. One model explains the Clemmsen's

Table 11.2 Weighted Proportion of Disabled Sample Persons Reporting Disabling Medical Conditions By Condition, 1984 National Long-Term Care Surkvey, by Sex

	IADL disability		1 to 2 ADLs disabilities		3 to 4 ADLs disabilities		5 to 6 ADLs disabilities		TOTAL	
	Males	Females	Males	Females	Males	Females	Males	Females	Males	Females
Cancer	4.6	3.3	4.8	3.3	7.2	5.3	8.3	7.4	5.7	4.2
Ischemic heart disease	5.8	3.4	2.4	3.2	5.1	4.4	8.0	4.5	5.0	3.6
Hypertension	7.4	10.2	6.0	9.7	6.2	13.7	5.9	11.6	6.6	10.8
Other circulatory disease	29.9	26.5	29.4	24.0	34.1	29.3	48.4	40.8	33.6	28.1
Diabetes	4.9	6.2	4.1	6.5	7.0	7.0	7.1	9.7	5.4	6.9
Senile Dementia	12.3	14.9	10.5	14.8	16.9	15.5	19.5	23.8	13.7	16.2
Mental disorders	3.7	4.1	4.3	4.2	3.4	5.8	5.5	6.2	4.1	4.7
Parkinson's	4.3	6.9	8.7	5.5	8.9	9.6	20.4	13.5	9.1	7.8
Visual disorders	17.4	16.5	17.8	13.3	14.3	14.5	13.3	13.0	16.4	14.6
Deafness	12.4	4.2	8.7	3.3	4.3	2.6	4.7	6.0	8.7	3.9
Ulcers	1.2	0.6	0.6	1.1	2.1	.07	0.9	0.5	1.2	0.8
Hernia	1.5	2.4	2.1	2.0	1.2	1.7	1.1	1.9	1.5	2.1
Other digestive disorders	4.4	3.9	3.4	4.4	4.4	4.0	4.9	4.9	4.2	4.2
Kidney & bladder disease	2.6	2.4	3.5	2.4	2.9	3.4	3.9	3.1	3.2	2.7
Genito-urinary disease	2.5	0.3	2.0	0.9	2.5	0.3	2.2	0.2	2.3	0.5

Emphysema & bronchitis	10.8	3.6	8.4	2.8	5.5	2.1	10.2	2.1	9.2	2.9
Acute respiratory disease	7.9	5.0	7.1	4.3	5.0	3.8	5.3	2.5	6.8	4.2
Skin disease	0.7	1.6	0.6	1.5	0.6	2.0	0.3	1.7	0.6	1.7
Arthritis	22.0	34.8	35.7	43.8	32.6	48.9	19.7	33.8	27.3	40.0
Other skeletal problems	17.8	19.8	26.8	25.7	35.0	27.5	22.3	19.7	23.8	23.1
Residual	4.1	15.5	8.4	17.8	12.7	21.4	6.1	20.2	7.0	17.9
Mean Number of Conditions	1.8	1.9	2.0	1.9	2.1	2.2	2.2	2.3	2.0	2.0

hook as due to the dependence of the tumor on hormonal changes (e.g., Moolgavkar et al., 1979; DeLisi, 1977). A second theory is that the "hook" is generated because there are *two* basic disease processes operating. The two-disease model is supported by the observation that the typically more aggressive premenopausal disease is related more strongly to a family history of breast cancer—suggesting a stronger genetic component for premenopausal disease.

To estimate the parameters of a two disease model, and to examine the biological significance of those parameters, we fit the 1969–1971 U.S. breast cancer mortality data for women using a form of equation (2) modified to represent the overall mortality risk from breast cancer as a product of two disease processes, or

$$\mu^*(a) = \sum_{j=1}^{2} \mu_j(a - l_j) \tag{13}$$

where μ_j is the population Weibull function (2) for the *j*th type of disease where the parameters are estimated separately for the two diseases. These hazards, when added together (13), best reproduce the age specific mortality rates. The fit obtained with the two disease model is presented in Figure 11.5.

The composite curve (C) fits the total breast cancer mortality curve quite well. Included in the figure are the curves for the two disease components. One curve (A) reaches a peak about menopause and then decreases. The second (B) shows a monotonic increase in risk with age. This is due to differences in the estimated parameters provided in Table 11.3.

We see that the heterogeneity parameter (3.86×10^{-3}) for disease type A (i.e., "premenopausal" disease) suggests a high degree of individual variation in risk. The different value of m (i.e., 7) for the premenopausal disease suggests that it is more rapidly onsetting than the postmenopausal disease (where m = 4) even though the rate of tumor growth (i.e., $l = 11.7$ years) is similar to that for "postmenopausal" disease.

The parameter values suggest the possibility that the Clemmsen's hook may be due to the rapid exhaustion (death) of persons with the premenopausal type of disease process in the population. The parameter estimates are consistent with data which show that the so-called "premenopausal" disease has strong genetic determinants (represented in the model by the value of *s*) with the relative risks for certain types of family pedigrees approaching 50 to 1 (Anderson, 1970, 1972, 1975). The estimates are also consistent with the finding that this type of disease is often due to a more aggressive cell type with poorer survival. More recently, clinical trials in Italy have identified strong

Figure 11.5 Observed and predicted single year of age probabilities of death due to breast cancer for white females in the U.S. in 1969. △, **observed probability of death caused by breast cancer; ◇, predicted probability of death caused by breast cancer; +, hypothesized probability of death caused by premenopausal disease; ×, hypothesized probability of death caused by postmenopausal disease.**

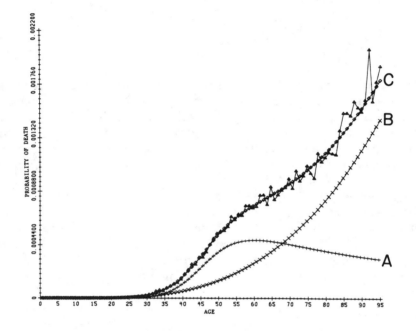

heterogeneity in breast cancer patients who are diagnosed at early ages in terms of the likelihood of micro-metastatic spread even when the primary tumor is diagnosed very early and resected nodes prove negative upon pathological examination. In the laboratory, markers of this subclass of tumor cell types are being developed (e.g., high DNA volume; high prevalence of certain oncogenes) to be used to identify individuals with this type of disease.

The second curve (B) shows little heterogeneity (i.e., $s_2 = \infty$) which is consistent with the weaker genetic linkage of late (i.e., "postmeno-pausal") breast cancer. This type of disease tends to be hormonally dependent (i.e., estrogen receptor positive) and have a less aggressive cell type.

These results show that, with detailed biological models of chronic disease processes fit to population data, certain types of biological models can be rejected. For example, a single disease, multihit model could not be made to fit the data in Figure 11.5. Nor could a two-

Table 11.3 Parameter Estimates of a Two-Disease Model of Breast Cancer Mortality Among White Females in the U.S., 1969

Premenopausal disease (A)	Postmenopausal disease (B)
$\bar{\alpha}_1 = 2.65 \times 10^{-13}$	$\bar{\alpha}_2 = 2.57 \times 10^{-9}$
$m_1 = 7.0^a$	$m_2 = 4.0^a$
$s_1 = 3.86 \times 10^{-3}$	$s_2 = \infty^a$
$l_1 = 11.61$	$l_2 = l_1{}^a$

[a] m_1, m_2, s_2 and l_2 are constrained parameters.

disease model with each disease being of the multihit type fit the data unless one disease was modeled as having strong individual variation. Within the set of models that do work, however, one must rely on biological data and theory to select between models. For example, the fact that epidemiological data show that certain subpopulations have a 50 to 1 risk is consistent with the heterogeneity parameter estimates for the premenopausal disease. The fact that women who manifest breast cancer premenopausally are a mixed group with very different prognoses and tumor cell characteristics is consistent with the findings in Figure 11.5 that show that there is a mixutre of the two disease types even at younger ages. Thus, the breast cancer analysis shows how population, epidemiological, clinical, and laboratory data and analyses can be used in a broad assessment of a sex-linked disease process.

Case Example: Lung Cancer

Our second example is lung cancer—which affects both males and females. We again employ the multistage/hit model of carcinogenesis as operationalized in equation (2). But in this analysis we will examine U.S. and Swedish cohort lung cancer mortality for the period 1950–1951 to 1981–1982. This allows us to examine cultural differences in sex specific cohort patterns where there were large differences in cohort exposures to certain risk factors. This occurred for lung cancer because, during World War II in Sweden, tobacco products were hard to get causing the early smoking experience of certain Swedish cohorts to be very different than their U.S. counterparts. Thus, the cohort specific differences in U.S. and Swedish smoking experience as a type of long-term natural experiment to asses the effect of that exogenous exposure (Manton, Malker, & Malker, 1986).

We found striking mortality differences for both male and female cohorts. These are illustrated in Figures 11.6a and 11.6b.

In the U.S., males currently have higher mortality rates but mortality increases for recent cohorts have stopped and apparently even begun to reverse (Manton et al., 1986). In contrast, the increases in mortality for recent U.S. female cohorts have been very rapid. The U.S. patterns may be compared to that for Swedish male and female cohorts that show (a) lower overall rates and (b) Swedish females manifesting only modest cohort increases.

The coefficients estimated for each of the models are presented in Table 11.4.

The latency times (k—the time from the initiation of the tumor to death) for both the U.S. and Swedish females are 2 to 4 years lower than for males. The $\bar{\alpha}_{30}$ values (the proportionality factor in equation (2)) represent the average lung cancer risk of a cohort at age 30. The ratio of the $\bar{\alpha}_{30}$ for two cohorts thus is a crude relative risk measure (adjusted for the age variation in risk reflected in the Weibull function). U.S. males have the highest level of risk—nearly twice that of Swedish male for the 1920 birth cohort. However, the rate of increase of that risk over cohorts is lowest for U.S. males—though similar (3.81) to Swedish males (4.2) and females (4.46). What is striking is the rapid increase in U.S. female lung cancer risks—rising 8.75 times between the 1885 and 1920 birth cohorts. The 1920 U.S. female cohort has over twice the lung cancer risks of Swedish females—though the 1885 U.S. and Swedish cohorts were nearly the same.

This example extends the breast cancer analysis by introducing a detailed analysis of cohort differences and the effects of a natural risk factor experiment—all premised on a biologically motivated model of the disease process.

Case Example: Stomach Cancer

A third type of model was used in an analysis of stomach cancer (Manton, Stallard, Burdick, & Tolley, 1979). This model allowed for age variation in the rate of growth of the tumors by generalizing the Weibull function as,

$$\mu(a) = \alpha(a - [l \cdot I^q])^{m-1} \tag{14}$$

Equation (14) allows a positive nonlinear correlation between the time to the onset of a tumor and its latency time—possibly due to a slower metabolic rate advanced ages. The application of the model to U.S. male and female stomach cancer data for 1975 produced the parameter estimates in Table 11.5

The parameters show that, under this model, there are biological similarities and differences in stomach cancer risks in U.S. males and females. The stomach cancer risk, governed by α, is 59% greater for males than females. Coefficients l and q govern the correlation of age

Figure 11.6A U.S. and Swedish sex specific lung cancer mortality rates: U.S. males and females.

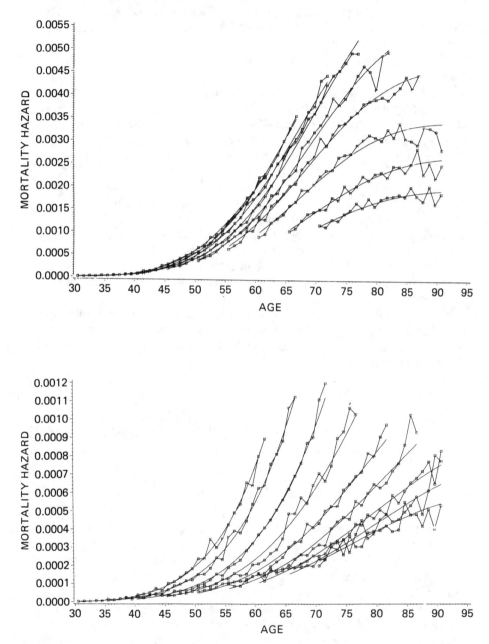

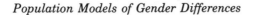

Figure 11.6B U.S. and Swedish sex specific lung cancer mortality rates: Swedish males and females.

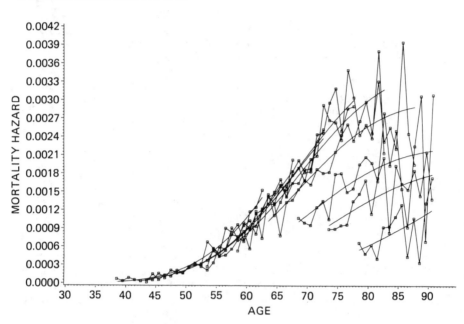

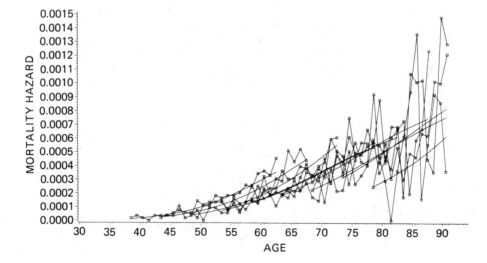

Table 11.4 Weibull Hazard Function Parameter Estimates for U.S. and Sweden: Lung Cancer Mortality

Year of birth	$\bar{\alpha}_{y_0}$		β_{y_0}	
	United States	Sweden	United States	Sweden
		Males		
1885	6.89×10^{-12}	3.45×10^{-12}	1.74×10^{-10}	1.11×10^{-10}[a]
	(2.29×10^{-13})	(9.52×10^{-13})	(1.06×10^{-11})	(6.08×10^{-11})
1890	1.07×10^{-11}	5.85×10^{-12}	2.17×10^{-10}	1.76×10^{-10}
	(2.93×10^{-13})	(1.30×10^{-12})	(9.78×10^{-12})	(6.56×10^{-11})
1895	1.32×10^{-11}	9.47×10^{-12}	1.96×10^{-10}	2.24×10^{-10}
	(3.44×10^{-13})	(1.91×10^{-12})	(8.47×10^{-12})	(6.84×10^{-11})
1900	1.50×10^{-11}	1.09×10^{-11}	1.79×10^{-10}	2.18×10^{-10}
	(4.03×10^{-13})	(2.26×10^{-12})	(8.54×10^{-12})	(7.03×10^{-11})
1905	1.73×10^{-11}	1.17×10^{-11}	1.65×10^{-10}	2.19×10^{-10}
	(4.90×10^{-13})	(2.16×10^{-12})	(9.66×10^{-12})	(8.34×10^{-11})
1910	2.02×10^{-11}	1.19×10^{-11}	2.21×10^{-10}	2.42×10^{-10}
	(6.23×10^{-13})	(2.91×10^{-12})	(1.54×10^{-11})	(1.17×10^{-10})
1915	2.27×10^{-11}	1.19×10^{-11}	2.38×10^{-10}	1.98×10^{-10}[a]
	(7.70×10^{-13})	(3.24×10^{-12})	(2.39×10^{-11})	(1.63×10^{-10})
1920	2.63×10^{-11}	1.45×10^{-11}	5.03×10^{-10}	2.30×10^{-10}[a]
	(1.01×10^{-12})	(4.45×10^{-12})	(5.67×10^{-11})	(3.05×10^{-10})
K	20.11	21.56		
m	6.0	6.0		
		Females		
1885	6.74×10^{-13}	6.38×10^{-13}	4.42×10^{-11}	2.48×10^{-11}[a]
	(3.81×10^{-14})	(1.48×10^{-13})	(6.38×10^{-12})	(2.24×10^{-11})
1890	7.87×10^{-13}	7.22×10^{-13}	4.42×10^{-11}	3.91×10^{-11}[a]
	(4.10×10^{-14})	(1.35×10^{-13})	(5.60×10^{-12})	(2.45×10^{-11})
1895	9.81×10^{-13}	9.64×10^{-13}	4.10×10^{-11}	6.01×10^{-11}
	(5.07×10^{-14})	(1.45×10^{-13})	(5.74×10^{-12})	(2.77×10^{-11})
1900	1.33×10^{-12}	1.19×10^{-12}	5.01×10^{-11}	1.00×10^{-10}
	(7.18×10^{-14})	(1.68×10^{-13})	(7.57×10^{-12})	(3.99×10^{-11})
1905	1.90×10^{-12}	1.23×10^{-12}	4.21×10^{-11}	1.08×10^{-10}
	(1.07×10^{-13})	(1.69×10^{-13})	(9.28×10^{-12})	(5.07×10^{-11})
1910	2.71×10^{-12}	1.38×10^{-12}	1.55×10^{-11}[a]	5.73×10^{-11}[a]
	(1.62×10^{-13})	(1.74×10^{-13})	(1.18×10^{-11})	(5.55×10^{-11})
1915	4.27×10^{-12}	1.97×10^{-12}	Ftn. b	1.50×10^{-10}[a]
	(2.80×10^{-13})	(2.81×10^{-13})		(1.20×10^{-10})
1920	5.90×10^{-12}	2.85×10^{-12}	1.07×10^{-11}[a]	3.60×10^{-10}[a]
	(4.32×10^{-13})	(4.46×10^{-13})	(4.34×10^{-11})	(2.58×10^{-10})
K	18.11	17.26		
m	6.0	6.0		

[a]Standard error was over half the size of the coefficient.
[b]Parameter was too small for precise estimation.

Table 11.5 Parameter Values for Latency Model Estimated over the Age Range 25 to 94: Both Sexes

	Male	Female
α	2.30×10^{-13}	1.44×10^{-13}
m	6.0	6.0
l	5.88×10^{-1}	1.03×10^{-1}
q	6.72×10^{-1}	1.19
ϕ	4.34×10^{-2}	4.28×10^{-2}
	$\chi^2 = 15.4$	$\chi^2 = 49.2$
Age	Male Latency	Female Latency
25	5.1	4.7
60	9.2	13.3
90	12.1	21.5

of tumor onset with rate of tumor growth. In Table 11.5, latency is similar for males and females at age 25; by age 90 it is 77% longer for females (i.e., 21.5 versus 12.1 years). Interestingly, ϕ, a parameter indicating the proportion of the population susceptible to stomach cancer, shows little differences in susceptibility for males and females.

Case Example: A Model of Carcinogenesis with Immunological Surveillance
An alternative cancer model was presented by Burch (1976). He argued that differences in immunological surveillance have to be represented in models of carcinogenesis. He does this by assuming that the tumor can only express itself if a given number of errors (say N) occur in stem cells in the immune system to permit mutated cells in the target organ to avoid being eliminated and thus initiate tumor growth. This produces the modified Weibull function,

$$\mu(a) = \frac{-\partial}{\partial a} \ln[1 - \{1 - \exp[-\alpha \, a^m/m]\}^N] \tag{15}$$

Such a model could be useful to explain sex differences in tumor risks if there is indeed a strong sex difference in the efficacy of the immunological system with regard to control of early neoplastic growth. Fits of this model to the same stomach cancer data as in the prior example showed that the model with the nonlinear correlation fit the data better. Naturally, the longer latency or tumor growth time for females in that model might also be interpreted as being due to a stronger immunological response for females—but at a difference stage of the disease process. That is, Burch's model reflects differences in the risk of the initiation of a tumor (i.e., a failure of immunological surveillance to identify mutated cells) while our model suggests that the slower growth may be due to a less favorable environment for tumor growth at later ages.

Finally, it is worthwhile to emphasize that the analysis of stomach cancer mortality rates for birth cohorts produced very different parameter estimates than for the analysis of cross-sectional data (e.g., Manton & Stallard, 1982). Using cohort data the m parameter was estimated to be two units smaller in cohort than in the cross-sectional data. This difference is due to the confounding of the within-cohort age trajectory of mortality risks with between-cohort differences. This confounding is strongest for disease processes with pronounced cohort differences such as stomach or lung cancer (though possibly not for, say, colon cancer). Nonetheless one still observed a strong slowing in the rate of increase of population stomach cancer mortality risks at advanced ages in the cohort analyses and strong differences in the trajectory of stomach cancer mortality risks for females for the two oldest cohorts.

Case Example: Total Mortality Differences at Advanced Ages

Another potential application of these models is to the analysis of total mortality differences at advanced ages. The results of an application of different population level Gompertz models to recent elderly Medicare cohorts are presented in Table 11.6 (Manton, Stallard, & Vaupel, 1986).

In Table 11.6, we compared sex differences in mortality in terms of the level of mortality, the degree of risk heterogeneity present in the population and the parameters controlling the rate of aging. For example, we compared the estimates of the Gompertz rate parameter (i.e., β in $\alpha e^{\beta t}$) under different assumptions about individual aging differences within cohort. The column marked "Homogeneous" represents the model which assumes that all persons in the cohort have *identical* rates of aging.

We also present estimates of the Gompertz aging function under two different assumptions of how individual differences in the rate of aging are distributed. The estimates of the Gompertz parameter are similar for the gamma and inverse Gaussian assumptions but both sets are quite different than for the homogeneous population model. The estimates for the homogeneous model are lower than what is usually assumed to be a biologically plausible value for $\beta \times 10^2$. The values when heterogeneity is assumed to exist, in contrast, are in a biologically reasonable range and furthermore, suggest significant declines in the rate of aging for the more recent cohorts—an observation consistent with recent increases in life expectancy at advanced ages, and the relative constancy in recent years of the mix of causes of death at

Table 11.6 Alternative Estimates of Gompertz Rate Parameter β under Three Marginal Distributions of Frailty, for Males

Cohort/age range	Gamma	$\beta \times 10^2$ Inverse Gaussian	"Homogeneous"
1902 65–75	7.34 (.10)	7.96 (.24)	6.26 (.06)
1900 67–77	7.38 (.11)	8.03 (.26)	6.11 (.06)
1898 69–79	7.73 (.12)	8.40 (.28)	6.26 (.06)
1896 71–81	7.88 (.14)	8.54 (.30)	6.18 (.06)
1894 73–83	8.20 (.15)	8.84 (.31)	6.22 (.06)
1892 75–85	8.65 (.18)	9.24 (.33)	6.32 (.06)
1890 77–87	9.14 (.21)	9.67 (.35)	6.44 (.07)
1888 79–89	9.48 (.24)	9.83 (.36)	6.34 (.07)
1886 81–91	9.81 (.28)	9.90 (.35)	6.17 (.08)
1884 83–93	10.29 (.32)	10.06 (.35)	6.09 (.09)

Note: Standard errors in given in parentheses.

advanced ages despite significant increases in the average age of death (for both males and females) for most of the major causes of death (Manton, 1985).

The model of mortality clearly suggests some slowing in the rate of aging among elderly persons in more recent cohorts (Jones, 1956). It is also useful to examine certain other biological implications of this effort at population modeling. In Table 11.7 we show how the coefficient of variation of individual aging rates changes under the two assumptions about the form of the distribution of these differences.

Under the gamma model the coefficient of variation is constant over age. For the inverse Gaussian it is declining. The gamma model thus suggests that heterogeneity of physiological status is preserved within

Table 11.7 Alternative Estimate of $\gamma^2(x)$, Age-Specific Squared Coefficient of Variation of Conditional Inverse Gaussian Frailty Distribution Based on α and β Parameter Estimates for the 1892 Birth Cohorts

	Males		Females	
Age	Gompertz	Weibull	Gompetz	Weibull
0	.443	.122	.662	.208
45	.430	.121	.653	.207
65	.375	.117	.597	.202
70	.347	.115	.561	.198
75	.313	.111	.511	.192
80	.275	.106	.449	.182
85	.236	.099	.381	.170
90	.198	.092	.312	.155
95	.163	.084	.249	.138
		Gamma Model		
	.211	.091	.288	.141
	[88.2]	[90.5]	[91.8]	[94.1]

Note: Values in brackets indicate ages at which $\gamma^2(x)$ for the inverse Gaussian model are the same values as for the Gamma model.

elderly cohorts while the inverse Gaussian model suggests it is decreasing. It is contrary to our conception of mortality at advanced ages as a balance between lethal thresholds or regions and decreasing ability to maintain homeostasis, for the risk heterogeneity of individuals to decrease so markedly at advanced ages. It is also contrary to existing studies of aging individuals, which show considerable heterogeneity among persons surviving into their eighties and beyond. It is then comforting that, in the population modeling effort, consistent with biological reasoning, the gamma model of individual differences provided a better fit to the Medicare population data than the inverse Gaussian model (Manton, Stallard, & Vaupel, 1986).

A Stochastic Process Model of Sex Differences in Mortality

Above we examined the application of biologically motivated models to population mortality data. Because of the limited amount of information on covariates in that data, the development of analytic models necessarily relied heavily on ancillary biological concepts and data. In this section we deal with data from longitudinally followed community populations. Because of the richness of the covariate information in that type of study we can estimate the parameters of more general models such described by equations (4) and (7). The examples we discuss involve data from both the first Duke Longitudinal Study and the Framingham Heart Study. Although having only 267 persons, the first Duke Longitudinal study included the extreme elderly (average age was 71.3 years at entry) who were closely monitored for over 21 years and had rich batteries of physiological and psychological variables assessed. The Framingham Heart Study population was much larger but younger (mean age at entry was 43 years), and had less extensive sets of risk factor and physiological variables measured.

Male and Female Differences in Survival and Risk Factor Changes

The application of our two-component model is very different from standard risk-factor assessments using Cox or logistic regression procedures. Cox and logistic regression procedures are not models of the underlying physiological processes. The coefficients in those functions represent the fixed contribution of a given covariate to the relative risk of the event over a specified time interval. In contrast, the coefficients of the multivariate stochastic process model described in equations (4) and (7) do represent the parameters of the basic physiological process. Because the parameter estimates reflect the operation of the process, to assess what the effect of physiological variable dynamics, lethal regions, or differences in the risk factor distribution represent in terms of sex differences in survival, male and female life tables can be calculated with equations (8) to (12). This is illustrated in Table 11.8 for Framingham males and females.

Both standard life table parameters (e.g., the surviving proportion, l_t, and the age specific life expectancy, $\overset{\circ}{e}_t$ and age specific means and standard deviations for nine risk factors are presented in Table 11.8. We see, for example, that the remaining life expectancy at age 30 is 43.75 years for males and 48.98 years for females based upon the male and female parameters estimated separately for the linear dynamic and quadratic mortality functions (i.e., equations (4) and (7)). At age 90 males have 2.85 years of life expectancy remaining—females have 3.55 years. In addition we see the risk factors and physiological parameters changing with age, for example, male vital capacity dropped from 140 at age 30 to 72 at age 100—females drop from 115 to 45. It also should be noted that the direction of change of the risk factors can change with age (e.g., diastolic blood pressure). Thus, the model does not limit functional changes to be linear, or even monotonic, because the interaction of dynamics and mortality can be modelled as non-linear across the age intervals.

These questions can also be used to examine changes in survival due to various types of risk factor and aging process interventions. These interventions can be modelled by altering the dynamic or mortality equation coefficients in a specified way. In Figure 11.7 we present the survival curve for males (curve A) and females (curve B) based on

Table 11.8 Estimated Cohort Survival (l_t), Life Expectancy Function (e^o_t), and Standard Deviations: Males and Females, Aged 30 Years, Framingham, Mass. Heart Study—Baseline Projection Model

t	l_t	e^o_t	AGE	PP	DPB	QI	CHOL	BLDSUG	HEMO	VITC	CIG
						MALES					
0	100,000	43.75	30	45.00	80.00	260.00	215.00	80.00	145.00	140.00	14.00
				13.70	12.53	34.43	41.42	29.64	10.25	18.87	11.53
10	98,203	34.45	40	41.18	83.18	271.87	241.20	78.56	147.91	138.04	14.96
				13.69	12.53	34.38	41.40	29.63	10.25	18.86	11.52
20	94,265	25.66	50	47.66	83.33	275.98	241.06	83.68	149.62	127.44	12.92
				13.69	12.52	34.30	41.38	29.62	10.24	18.80	11.51
30	85,912	17.61	60	55.27	83.25	273.36	233.03	90.94	150.40	114.30	9.34
				13.68	12.50	34.12	41.33	29.60	10.24	18.80	11.49
40	68,018	10.77	70	62.98	82.80	266.10	223.01	98.52	150.73	100.82	4.91
				13.65	12.46	33.76	41.22	29.57	10.22	18.71	11.46
50	35,334	5.80	80	70.39	82.00	257.22	213.18	105.74	150.95	88.40	0.00
				13.60	12.39	33.06	40.99	29.49	10.20	18.54	0.00
60	5,754	2.85	90	77.33	80.84	250.34	204.70	111.86	151.90	78.00	0.00
				13.50	12.23	31.78	40.57	29.31	10.07	18.07	0.00
70	55	1.55	100	83.35	79.56	249.14	197.19	116.78	153.60	71.51	0.00
				13.33	11.95	29.97	39.81	29.01	9.99	17.51	0.00

FEMALES

Values shown as mean (standard deviation).

Age	Survivors	Life exp.	Age	PP	DBP	QI	CHOL	BLDSUG	HEMO	VITC	CIG
0	100,000	48.98	30	45.00 (15.52)	75.00 (12.27)	235.00 (44.67)	200.00 (42.87)	80.00 (22.14)	125.00 (10.21)	115.00 (17.03)	8.00 (8.13)
10	98,702	39.55	40	40.07 (15.52)	78.33 (12.27)	248.76 (44.66)	233.34 (42.85)	77.46 (22.14)	130.76 (10.20)	116.86 (17.02)	10.02 (8.12)
20	96,360	30.37	50	48.89 (15.52)	80.00 (12.27)	256.63 (44.63)	246.18 (42.82)	81.91 (22.44)	135.39 (10.20)	105.68 (17.02)	10.13 (8.11)
30	91,882	21.58	60	58.90 (15.51)	81.66 (12.26)	256.81 (44.57)	252.16 (42.76)	88.05 (22.13)	138.92 (10.20)	91.93 (17.01)	8.92 (8.10)
40	81,230	13.66	70	68.79 (15.51)	82.95 (12.25)	252.49 (44.44)	255.92 (42.62)	94.19 (22.11)	141.79 (10.19)	78.08 (16.98)	6.77 (8.07)
50	55,236	7.44	80	78.25 (15.49)	83.77 (12.22)	244.53 (44.17)	259.34 (42.32)	99.93 (22.07)	144.18 (10.17)	64.96 (16.92)	4.03 (8.00)
60	15,993	3.55	90	86.93 (15.44)	83.93 (12.17)	234.72 (43.59)	263.61 (41.71)	105.08 (22.00)	146.08 (10.13)	53.45 (16.80)	1.13 (7.87)
70	442	1.76	100	94.31 (15.36)	83.18 (12.05)	226.31 (42.26)	269.59 (40.56)	109.56 (21.84)	147.38 (9.89)	45.06 (16.56)	0.00 (0.00)

Median age: 75.98

PP = Pulse pressure (mm Hg); DBP = Diastolic blood pressure (mm Hg); QI = Quetelet index; CHOL = Cholesterol (mg/dl); BLDSUG = Blood sugar; HEMO = Hemoglobin; VITC = Vital Capacity Index (cl/m^2); CIG = number of cigarettes per day.

Figure 11.7 Baseline and predicted survival curves for males and females.

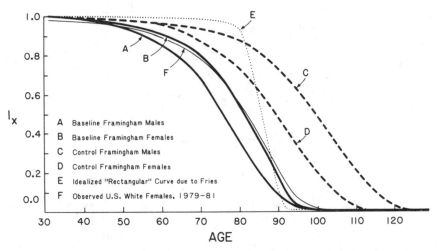

conditions as observed in Framingham, and the survival curve for Framingham males and females when the age dynamics and variability of risk factors are controlled (curves C and D respectively).

In addition to the Framingham results, we also plotted the idealized "rectangular" survival curve based on estimates due to Fries (1980, 1983) (curve E) and the observed U.S. white female survival curve for 1979–1981 (curve F). None of the empirical survival curves have the same shape as the Fries theoretical "rectangularized" curve with the empirically derived curves manifesting much greater variability. These curves imply that mortality does not increase as rapidly at advanced ages as for the Fries curve with more females *observed* in 1979–1981 (curve F) to survive to advanced ages than was projected under the Fries model for ideal conditions (see Schneider and Guralnik, 1987). Recently Fries (1987) has changed his model of mortality compression by suggesting that the standard deviation for the age at death distribution is seven, rather than four, years (see Fries 1980, 1983). This change is not, however, based on a clear theoretical argument and is an empirical adjustment to allow his theoretical curves to at least match current data.

The change in survival curves for Framingham males and females (C and D) show expected increases in life expectancy with the maintenance of the risk factors in clinically desirable ranges at advanced ages. It is of interest that the values of physiological variables for centenarians tend to be similar to those found at much earlier ages.

Under these interventions life expectancy at age 30 increased roughly 24 and 8 years (to 67 years and 57 years) for males and females respectively, with far more persons expected to live to advanced ages than under the Fries model. The fact that males derive more benefit from intervention in these chronic disease risk factors is not surprising because (a) most of the community epidemiological studies focused on identifying chronic disease risks for middle aged males, and (b) the apparently strong role of autoimmune, hormonal and neurological factors (which were not assessed in the Framingham study) in female mortality risks at advanced ages. In addition, the interventions were based on the assumption that initial risk factor values should not be allowed to change with age. Though this strategy appears reasonable for males, it is not an optimal assumption for females. For example, we know that risk factor changes and their association with disease risks is apparently strongly affected by hormonal factors that change at menopause. Thus, the "optimal" control of these risk factors for females will change with age, requiring a more complex model than we have attempted to construct here.

In applying this model there are a number of features in addition to risk-factor dynamics that are of biological interest. For example, because the risk factors are multiplied by a Gompertz function, the dependence of mortality risks on age can be estimated *net* of the effects of the observed risk factors and their changes with age. Thus, in contrast to cause elimination life-table strategies and standard risk factor analyses there is a biologically motivated age-dependent force of mortality that is independent of a specific disease. It is interesting to note that the Gompertz function really represents an "age" residual for mortality risks. Thus, as more dimensions of aging and mortality processes are made explicit as dimensions of the model, the effect of the Gompertzian dynamics of "senescence" will decline. Consequently, one can also simulate the effects of cause elimination (i.e., synthetically altering the mortality risk of one or more disease processes)—but more realistically than in the standard model of such adjustments as the different causes interact by being dependent on a common set of physiological variables and a common age-dependent Gompertz function. These *dependent* competing risk effects (Assumption 2) and the independent competing risk effects (Assumption 3), as well as the baseline life table values (Assumption 1) are illustrated for both nonsmoking males and females in the Framingham Heart Study in Table 11.9.

Life expectancy increases less under the elimination of cardiovascular disease in this model (i.e., for males at age 80, 11.10 for dependent competing risks versus 12.16 years for independent competing risks) because more persons with adverse risk factor levels survive to advanced ages (e.g., at age 90 after the elimination of heart disease, blood sugar levels for males rise from 111.83 to 114.98 mg/dl because persons with high blood sugar levels live longer without the risk of heart disease).

This type of analysis of age changes in the effects of risk factors adjusted for dependent competing risks gives us considerably more insight into the mechanisms by which risk factors affect mortality. For example, at advanced ages the ability to maintain a moderately high Q.I. appears protective, e.g., elimination of cardiovascular disease among males drops the Q.I. at age 100 to 232.63 (from 249.21) indicating a strong selection against low Q.I. values by cardiovascular disease at advanced ages. The effect of such dependency between cardiovascular and other diseases increases with age—most notably above age 80. For females, because of their greater life expectancy the effects of dependency are deferred to much later ages than for males.

Sex Specific Analyses of Coronary Heart Disease Mortality

To further illustrate the use of these models in studying gender differences for specific chronic disease risks we will discuss results on Coronary Heart Disease (CHD) morbidity from a limited study of 10 years of follow-up in the Framingham Heart Study. In that anlaysis we examined both sex differences in the dynamics of a limited set of risk factors (age, pulse pressure, diastolic blood pressure, serum cholesterol, uric acid) and in the risk functions for CHD.

In the dynamic equations (Woodbury, Manton, & Stallard, 1981) we found sex differences in both the constant term *and* in the rate of age change in the risk factors. In those equations, *after* adjusting for measurement error and the effects of other covariates, the initial risk factor levels were slightly lower for females but showed faster age rates of increase. In the hazard equations, the linear effects for pulse pressure, diastolic blood pressure, and age were significant for both sexes while the linear terms for cholesterol and uric acid were significant only for males. There were far stronger nonlinear (quadratic effects) for pulse pressure, diastolic blood pressure, cholesterol, and uric acid for males.

In Figure 11.8 we present, for selected conditions for males and females, the probability of surviving from age 30 to 110 without a CHD event among all persons who survive to each age.

Up to age 60 there is a more rapid rate of decline in the proportion of males free of CHD than for females under "baseline" conditions. This is consistent with evidence on the early protective effects of female hor-

Table 11.9 Estimated Cohort Survival Function (l_x), Life Expectancy Function (e_t^o), and Risk Factor Means for Framingham Heart Study Males and Females Who are Nonsmokers Under Three Assumptions: (1) Baseline Values, (2) Eliminating Cardiovascular Disease (Dependent Competing Risks), and (3) Eliminating Cardiovascular Disease (Independent Competing Risks)

t Years Past 30)	Assumption Type	l_t	e_t^o	AGE	PP	DPB	QI	CHOL	BLDSUG	HEMO	VITC
						MALES					
0	1	100,000	45.32	30	45.00	80.00	260.00	215.00	80.00	145.00	140.00
	2	100,000	55.02		45.00	80.00	260.00	215.00	80.00	145.00	140.00
	3	100,000	55.89		45.00	80.00	260.00	215.00	80.00	145.00	140.00
10	1	98,681	35.86	40	40.42	83.30	272.42	241.33	79.60	146.25	140.71
	2	99,444	45.30		40.43	83.31	272.46	241.36	79.62	146.26	140.71
	3	99,444	46.18		40.42	83.30	272.42	241.33	79.60	146.25	140.71
20	1	95,722	26.79	50	46.81	83.44	277.11	241.50	84.61	148.03	130.87
	2	98,299	35.76		46.82	83.46	277.25	241.60	84.66	148.03	130.87
	3	98,301	36.65		46.81	83.44	277.11	241.50	84.61	148.03	130.87
30	1	89,023	18.38	60	54.56	83.36	274.83	233.57	91.62	149.19	117.42
	2	98,615	26.61		54.62	83.42	275.00	233.76	91.78	149.19	117.34
	3	95,626	27.51		54.56	83.36	274.83	233.57	91.62	149.19	117.42
40	1	73,070	11.15	70	62.51	82.90	267.49	223.51	98.91	150.01	103.05
	2	88,909	18.18		62.75	83.06	267.21	223.80	99.38	149.96	102.59
	3	88,982	19.14		62.51	82.90	267.49	223.51	98.91	150.01	103.05

Table 11.9 (continued)

50	1	40,044	5.87	80	70.22	82.04	258.04	213.53	105.79	150.80	89.37
	2	72,079	11.10		70.98	82.43	255.75	213.95	107.08	150.58	87.71
	3	72,712	12.16		70.22	82.04	258.04	213.53	105.79	150.80	89.37
60	1	6,697	2.86	90	77.31	80.86	250.65	204.74	111.83	151.91	78.18
	2	38,761	6.03		79.29	81.70	243.16	205.66	114.98	151.38	73.62
	3	41,872	7.18		77.31	80.86	250.65	204.74	111.83	151.91	78.18
70	1	65	1.55	100	83.35	79.57	249.21	197.13	116.78	153.59	71.53
	2	7,033	3.11		87.74	81.06	232.63	200.40	123.60	152.48	61.62
	3	11,213	4.24		83.35	79.57	249.21	197.13	116.78	153.59	71.53

FEMALES

0	1	100,000	49.85	30	45.00	75.00	235.00	200.00	80.00	125.00	115.00
	2	100,000	57.26		45.00	75.00	235.00	200.00	80.00	125.00	115.00
	3	100,000	57.71		45.00	75.00	235.00	200.00	80.00	125.00	115.00
10	1	98,845	40.37	40	39.82	78.53	250.19	233.36	76.70	128.15	118.33
	2	99,173	47.69		39.82	78.53	250.18	233.35	76.69	128.15	118.33
	3	99,174	48.15		39.82	78.53	250.19	233.36	76.70	128.15	118.33
20	1	96,857	31.08	50	48.57	80.22	258.81	246.53	80.84	132.43	107.69
	2	97,795	38.29		48.57	80.22	258.81	246.53	80.83	132.43	107.70
	3	97,796	38.75		48.57	80.22	258.81	246.53	80.84	132.43	107.69

30	1	93,013	22.14	60	58.61	81.93	260.71	252.75	87.01	136.18	93.97
	2	95,335	29.13		58.63	81.94	260.73	252.75	87.01	136.19	93.93
	3	95,337	29.61		58.61	81.93	260.71	252.75	87.01	136.18	93.97
40	1	83,321	14.04	70	68.61	83.26	257.05	256.67	93.38	139.59	79.81
	2	90,091	20.50		68.72	83.33	257.03	256.60	93.44	139.62	79.60
	3	90,111	21.00		68.61	83.26	257.05	256.67	93.38	139.59	79.81
50	1	58,136	7.66	80	78.21	84.10	249.26	260.14	98.48	142.72	66.15
	2	77,385	12.93		78.59	84.33	248.92	259.78	99.74	142.81	65.38
	3	77,588	13.47		78.21	84.10	249.26	260.14	98.48	142.72	66.15
60	1	17,867	3.66	90	87.04	84.27	239.14	264.22	105.08	145.46	53.95
	2	49,376	7.13		88.18	84.93	237.67	263.05	105.95	145.69	51.68
	3	50,592	7.72		87.04	84.27	239.14	264.22	105.08	145.46	53.95
70	1	539	1.76	100	94.48	83.44	229.05	269.57	109.90	147.50	44.88
	2	13,147	3.52		97.40	85.04	224.85	266.86	112.28	148.02	39.19
	3	15,660	4.12		94.48	83.44	229.05	269.57	109.90	147.50	44.88

PP = Pulse pressure (mm Hg); DBP = Diastolic blood pressure (mm Hg); QI = Quetelet index; CHOL = Cholesterol (mg/dl); BLDSUG = Blood sugar; HEMO = Hemoglobin; VITC = Vital Capacity Index (cl/m^2).

**Figure 11.8 Temporal changes in proportion of males surviving to *t*
based on three conditions: male and female baseline, with female linear
coefficients, and with fixed ideal blood pressure values.**

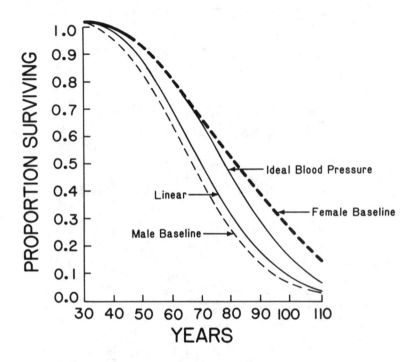

monal factors on CHD risks. Up to age 60 the rate of decline in the
survivability of the risk of CHD onset is very slow. After age 60 the
rate of decline for both males and females seems to stabilize, possibly
providing evidence of an acceleration of the decline in the proportion of
females without such disease at very advanced ages where female
protection by hormonal factors have diminished after menopause.

With the sex specific estimates of the dynamic and hazard functions,
one can explore variations in sex differences in disease and mortality
risks dynamically over the full life span by making changes in those
functions. For example, in Figure 11.8 we also plotted (a) the CHD
curve for males with blood pressure fixed at a clinically defined "ideal"
level and (b) the male curve with the linear terms from the female
hazard function substituted in the male hazard function. The second
condition shows the sensitivity of the male hazard to a redefinition of
the "lethal" region for CHD, that is, because we are *not* altering risk

factor variables or their dynamics—only the hazard function. Note that the substitution of the female linear terms in the male hazard function produces stronger reductions in risk at earlier ages because, at more advanced ages, the stronger quadratic male effects dominate. Thus, even at the same risk factor level and with the same risk factor dynamics, males have higher risks than females. This is consistent with our earlier descriptive results that suggest greater female "robustness" to certain cardiovascular risk factors—and it illustrates the effect in dynamic terms.

The Framingham experience described above is limited by short follow-up (10 years) and a low mean age at study entry (43 years). A comparison of these results (Woodbury & Manton, 1983) with those in the Duke Longitudinal Study (mean age at entry 71.3 years; mean age at 21 years of follow-up, 86 years) would suggest something of broader age changes in risk factor dynamics and mortality (Manton & Woodbury, 1983). Succinctly, the changes in that older cohort seem consistent with the trends discussed above. The age by sex interaction terms in the dynamic equations that were significant in the younger cohort were not significant at these advanced ages—though there were still differences in the risk factor means with females now being slightly *elevated*. In contrast, the hazard functions were quite different between the sexes—and very different from those estimated in the younger cohort. First, the constant hazard was much higher for males while the different quadratic coefficients tended to be less significant for males than for females. These changes from the younger cohort suggest difficulties in estimating the effects of individual risk factors against such a high male background hazard. This difficulty was one of the factors that led us to respecify the quadratic hazard with the Gompertz component.

The above results are suggestive of some differences in the age dependence of circulatory degenerative processes between males and females. Furthermore, part of the difference seems related to age specific factors not directly reflected by the available risk factors (e.g., hormonal shifts at menopause) but which have to be inferred from the population age dynamics of the risk factors, mortality, and morbidity risks for males and females.

SUMMARY

In this chapter we reviewed both models of sex differences in mortality and morbidity at later ages and presented some illustrative examples of the application of such models carried out with various types of population data. The illustrations show that biologically meaningful inferences can be made with population data if the analytic models employed are designed to be biologically "meaningful," that is, their construction is designed to reflect insights from ancillary biological data and theory.

From those analyses, though illustrative, we developed several insights into sex differences in the age dependence and interrelation of morbidity, disability, and mortality processes. Most basic perhaps, were the finding that females' greater prevalence of functional impairment was not due to differences in incidence but due to females' greater survival at any level of impairment at any age. The female survival advantage across impairment level and age seemed to result from sex differences in the type of diseases that were most often reported as causing disability. Males tended to be at higher risk of cancer, heart disease, and other disease processes that were relatively rapid in causing death. Females, in contrast, seemed to have higher risks of chronic degenerative processes (e.g., arthritis, Alzheimer's; osteoporosis) that progressed more slowly with death frequently resulting from chronic sequelae of the basic disease process after several years spent with that process. Frequently, these chronic degenerative diseases seemed to have a foundation in autoimmunological responses—a finding consistent with laboratory confirmed sex differences in immunological response. It was also notable that females had a high prevalence of certain factors (e.g., hypertension, diabetes, obesity) that are often viewed as risk factors for acute circulatory disease events. It suggests that the hormonal factors that appear to protect females from initiation of significant circulatory degeneration up to menopause are more powerful than exposure to these significant risk factors.

These findings could be examined in greater detail in data from epidemiological studies in which risk factors are assessed at multiple points in time. The application of a detailed two component model of human aging and mortality to these data show that intervention in the well-known chronic disease risk factors have a greater effect on male, than female, life expectancy. We also saw that the rate of age increase of female CHD risks were relatively low up to age 60 and then started to increase for females at later ages. It is clear, however, that even at advanced ages risk factors other than those for cancer and heart disease were operational for females—a finding consistent with the higher risks of autoimmune and other degenerative processes among females. These findings are suggestive of needed areas of investigation for understanding gender differences in morbidity, mortality, and disability processes using biologically detailed population models.

GLOSSARY OF SELECTED STATISTICAL AND DEMOGRAPHIC TERMS

Competing Risks—Risks that represent the fact that, in any given data set, the observation of certain events (e.g., death from cancer at a given age) will prevent the observation of other events (e.g., the age at which the person who died from cancer would have died from heart disease). If the risks of these events are not correlated then we have independent competing risks. If they are correlated (and there are many possible mechanisms to generate such correlations, such as a risk factor that affects the risk of death from two or more causes) then we have dependent competing risks.

Gamma Distribution—This is a type of long-tailed distribution that has been used to describe the distribution of "frailty" (e.g., the risk of death) in a population. It is used because it is a very flexible distribution that can approximate a wide range of other distributions. The form of the gamma distribution is determined by the values of two parameters—one is called the scale parameter and one is called the shape parameter. In the gamma distribution, in contrast to the normal distribution, these parameters are correlated and jointly determine the mean and variance of the distribution. An alternative distribution used for this purpose in modeling individual heterogeneity is the inverse Gaussian distribution.

Hazard Function—This is an equation that relates increases in the rate at which an event occurs in the population with age or time. Covariates may also be introduced in a hazard function in an effort to relate parts of the increased risk to more substantively meaningful variables than chronological age.

Gompertz Function—This is a specifc type of hazard function developed long ago (1825) by an actuary named Benjamin Gompertz. This specific hazard function is thought to well describe the age increase of mortality between ages 30 to 80. It has been used in many models of the human biology of aging and mortality (e.g., Strehler, 1977).

Grade of Membership Analysis—Is a type of multivariate analyses in which both regression functions and groupings of cases are determined from multivariate categorical data. The model is named after the coefficient used to describe how each case is related to each group defined by the model. Because a person may be a partial member of a group he may actually possess degrees or Grades of Membership in more than one group.

Life Table—This is a probability model for describing the age distribution of the risk-discrete events like mortality. It is composed of a number of different types of parameters that describe either the age-specific risks of events, or the risk of events over the life time remaining after a given age.

Logistic Regression—This is a type of regression often used in health studies because it describes how the risk of a discrete event is related to covariates. To model the probability of an outcome, and to obtain coefficients that produce a probability constrained to be between 0 and 1, the probability is modeled as a logistic function that is the natural logarithm of the "odds ratio" (i.e., p/1–p). Often the logistic function is misapplied because its highly nonlinear nature is not fully taken into account in interpreting results.

Quadratic Function—This is a type of hazard function or model (in addition to the Gompertz and Weibull models) that includes the effects of measured covariates. It models the risk of an event in terms of a constant effect and the linear, quadratic, and interactive effects of the covariates. This function is also useful for describing human aging changes and mortality in that it implies that there are physiological homeostatic (i.e., restorative) forces that cause mortality to increase in either direction from physiologically optimal values of the risk factors.

Random Walk Models—These are mathematical descriptions in which the change in the characteristics of a person is affected by random shocks. Usually, a random walk is viewed in terms of discrete changes. However, the importance of the random walk is that it describes the basic probability model from which the properties of many more complex stochastic processes can be determined.

Regression—This refers to equations that describe how an outcome event varies as a function of certain prior events or inputs. Such equations may be written in many different forms. They may be linear or nonlinear. They may describe dependence over time. They are a frequently used tool in statistical analyses. When the coefficients in the regression are related to the parameters of a process then the regression becomes a substantively interpretable model rather than simply being a parsimonious description of data.

Weibull Function—This is a type of hazard function used in models of human aging and mortality. Whereas the Gompertz function assumes that a person accumulates "wear" as a linear function of age, the Weibull function is premised on a number of discrete pathological changes (e.g., loss of specific types of functions) being accumulated over time.

REFERENCES

Anderson, D. E. (1970). Genetic considerations in breast cancer. In *Breast Cancer: Early and late*. Chicago: Chicago Year Book Medical Publishers.

Anderson, D. E. (1972). A genetic study of human breast cancer. *J National Cancer Inst, 48*, 1029–1034.

Anderson, D. E. (1975). Familial susceptibility. In J. F. Fraumeni (Ed.), *Persons at high risk of cancer*. New York: Academic Press

Archambeau, J. O., M. B., Heller, A. Akanuma, & D. Lubell, (1970). Biologic and clinical implications obtained from the analysis of cancer growth curves. *Clinical Obstetric Gynecology, 13*, 831–856.

Armitage, P., & R. Doll, (1954). The age distribution of cancer and a multistage theory of carcinogenesis. *British Journal of Cancer, 8*, 12.

Armitage, P., & R. Doll, (1961). Stochastic models for carcinogenesis. In J. Neyman (Ed.), *Proceedings of the fourth Berkeley symposium on mathematical statistics and probability, vol IV, biology and problems of health* (pp. 19–38). Berkeley: University of California Press.

Beckman, L., Singer, B., & Manton, K. G. (1989). Black/white differences in health status and mortality among the elderly. *Demography, 26*(4), 661–678.

Burch, P. R. J. (1976), *The biology of cancer: A new approach*. Baltimore: University Park Press.

Cook, P. J., Fellingham, S. A., & Doll, R. (1969). A mathematical model for the age distribution of cancer in man. *International Journal of Cancer, 4*, 93–112.

DeWaard, F., Baanders-VanHalewijn, E. A., & Huizinga, J. (1964). The bimodal age distribution of patients with mammary carcinoma. *Cancer, 17*, 141–151.

DeLisi, C. (1977). The age incidence of female breast cancer: Simple models and analysis of epidemiological patterns. *Math Biosc, 37*, 245–266.

Economos, A. C. (1982). Rate of aging, rate of dying, and the mechanisms of mortality. *Archives of Gerontological Geriatrics, 1*, 3–27.

Fries, J. F. (1980). Aging, natural death, and the compression of morbidity. *New England Journal of Medicine, 303*, 130–135.

Fries, J. F. (1983). The compression of morbidity. *Milbank Memorial Fund Quarterly, 61*, 397–419.

Fries, J. F. (1987). Reduction of the national morbidity. *Gerontologica Perspecta, 1*, 54–64.

Gillespie, D. T. (1983). The mathematics of simple random walks. *Naval Research News, 35*, 46–52.

Jaquez, J. A. (1972). *Compartmental analysis in biology and medicine*. Amsterdam: Elsevier.

Jones, H. B. (1956). A special consideration of the aging process, disease and life expectancy. *Adv Bio Med Phys, 4*, 281–337.

Knudson, A. G., Strong, L. C., & Anderson, D. E. (1973). Heredity and cancer in man. *Prog Med Genet, 9*, 113–158.

MacMahon, B., Cole, P., & Brown, J. (1973). Etiology of human breast cancer: A review. *Journal of the National Cancer Institute, 50,* 21–42.

Manton, K. G. (1985). Future patterns of chronic disease incidence, disability, and mortality among elderly. *NY State J Med, 85* (11), 623–633.

Manton, K. G. (1988a). Multistate models in health status forecasting. In F. J. Willekens (Ed.), *Multistate Demography: New Methods and Applications.* Amsterdam: D. Reidel.

Manton, K. G. (1988b). A longitudinal study of functional change and mortality in the United States. *Journal of Gerontology, 43,* 153–161.

Manton, K. G., Malker, H., & Malker, B. (1986). Comparison of temporal changes in U.S. and Swedish lung cancer, 1950–51 to 1981–82. *Journal of the National Cancer Institute, 77* (3), 665–675.

Manton, K. G., & Stallard, E. (1979). Maximum likelihood estimation of a stochastic compartment model of cancer latency: Mortality among white females. *Comput Biomed Res, 12,* 313–325.

Manton, K. G., & Stallard, E. (1981). Methods for evaluating the heterogeneity of aging processes in human populations using vital statistics data: Explaining the black/white mortality crossover by a model of mortality selection. *Human Biology, 53* (1), 47–67.

Manton, K. G., & Stallard, E. (1982). A population-based model of respiratory cancer incidence, progression, diagnosis, treatment and mortality. *Computers and Biomedical Research, 15,* 342–360.

Manton, K. G., Stallard, E., Burdick, D., & Tolley, H. D. (1979). A stochastic compartment model of stomach cancer with correlated waiting time distributions. *International Journal of Epidemiology, 8* (3), 283–291.

Manton, K. G., Stallard, E., & Poss, S. (1980). Estimates of U.S. multiple cause life tables. *Demography, 16* (2), 313–327.

Manton, K. G., Stallard, E., & Vaupel, J. W. (1986). Alternative models for the heterogeneity of mortality risks among the aged. *Journal of the American Statistical Association, 81,* 635–644.

Manton, K. G., & Woodbury, M. A. (1983). A Mathematical model of the physiological dynamics of aging and correlated mortality selection. II. Application to the Duke Longitudinal Study. *Journal of Gerontology, 38,* 406–413.

Manton, K. G., & Woodbury, M. A. (1985). A continuous-time multivariate Gaussian stochastic process model of change in discrete and continuous state variables. In N. Tuma (Ed.), *Sociological methodology* (pp. 277–315). San Francisco: Jossey Bass.

Matis, J. H., & Wehrly, T. E. (1979). Stochastic models of compartmental systems. *Biometrics, 35,* 199–220.

Moolgavkar, S. H., Stevens, R. G., & Lee, J. A. (1979). Effect of age on incidence of breast cancer in females. *J. National Cancer Institute, 62* 493–501.

Peto, R., Roe, F. J., Lee, P. N., et al. (1975). Cancer and aging in mice and men. *British Journal of Cancer, 32,* 411–425.

Sacher, G. A. (1977). Life table modification and life prolongation. In J. Birren & C. Finch (Eds.), *Handbook of the biology of aging* pp. 582–638. New York: Van Nostrand Reinhold.

Sacher, G. A., & Trucco, E. (1962). The stochastic theory of mortality. *Annals of the New York Academy of Sciences, 96,* 985.

Schneider, E. L., & Guralnik, J. M. (1987). The compression of morbidity: A dream that may come true someday! *Gerontologica Perspecta, 1,* 8–13.

Strehler, B. L. (1977). *Time, Cells and Aging.* New York: Academic Press.

Watson, G. (1977). Age incidence curves for cancer. *Proceedings of the National Academy of Sciences, 74,* 1341–1342.

Whittemore, A. S. (1977). The age distribution of human cancer for carcinogenic exposures of varying intensity. *American Journal of Epidemiology, 106,* 418–432.

Woodbury, M. A., & Manton, K. G. (1977). A random walk model of human mortality and aging. *Theoretical Population Biology, 11*(1), 37–48.

Woodbury, M. A., & Manton, K. G. (1983). A mathematical model of the physiological dynamics of aging and correlated mortality selection. I. Theoretical development and critiques. *Journal of Gerontology, 38,* 398–405.

Woodbury, M. A., Manton, K. G., & Stallard, E. (1981). A dynamic analysis of chronic disease development: A study of sex specific changes in coronary heart disease incidence and risk factors in Framingham. *International Journal of Epidemiology, 10*(4), 355–366.

End Notes: Closing the Gender Gap? Need for Future Research

Marcia G. Ory
Huber R. Warner

THE UNCERTAINTY OF GENDER GAP PREDICTIONS

Several gender differences in biology, behavior, and social roles have been documented in the preceding chapters. The impact of these differences on health and quality of life have also been explored. Yet, two major questions remain unanswered: Will the gender gap persist in the future? And what particular form will it take? While most researchers predict that there will be some narrowing of the gap, there is mixed opinion as to whether this will be due to men's adoption of healthier lifestyles, or to women's increased participation in less healthy behaviors and roles. For example, the changing sex ratio of deaths due to lung cancer between 1950 and 1980 can be attributed to increases in women's smoking relative to men's.

Nevertheless, future predictions are complicated by the complexity of factors contributing to gender differences in health and longevity, and by the lack of critical knowledge. More research is needed to understand how risk factors are changing over time and the contribution of changing risk factors on reported gender differentials. Two secular trends are worth further study: (1) women's tendency to engage in riskier behaviors and lifestyles, and (2) men's (at least those with high educational levels) recent predilection for healthier life-styles in the area of nutrition and exercise.

Unpredictable cohort changes in health and behavior also add to our uncertainties about future gender differentials. We cannot predict the consequences of the introduction of new fatal acute conditions such as

AIDS, which may affect one gender more than another. Or the effect of the dramatic increase in violence that is becoming more prevalent in certain subgroups of the male population.

DIRECTIONS FOR FUTURE RESEARCH

Research reported in this volume has shown that the sex mortality ratio differs by age group—with mortality rates for men and women becoming more similar in old age. This leads to some interesting questions about whether biological and social risk factors have different potency levels at different points in the life course. A life-course perspective is important for determining whether or not there are critical periods of susceptibility for different risk factors.

Additionally, the long latency period of many fatal chronic conditions may permit changes in survival patterns based on new medical advances. Little is known about whether the gender difference in longevity reflects sex differences in disease etiology or sex differences in survivorship.

There is also some speculation that men and women may have a differential response to the same risk factor. For example, men may be more susceptible than women to the influence of smoking on heart disease based on underlying biological differences. It will be important to assess the meaning and impact of particular risk factors for each sex.

While most previous research has focused on sex differences in mortality, more recent research is beginning to focus on differences in morbidity, functioning, and quality of life. While harder to assess in large scale studies, these are the areas that could be studied further to understand the day-to-day experience of men and women's lives. Especially neglected, and begging for attention, are studies of gender differences in the health and functioning of special populations that have traditionally been overlooked—the oldest old, racial, and ethnic minorities, and those living in rural areas.

Several methodological difficulties in examining and interpreting gender differences are discussed throughout the volume. The failure to include both biological and social variables in the same study is cited as a major problem that can only be solved through much needed interdisciplinary research. While scientifically rewarding, interdisciplinary research is not always easy. It requires scientists who can work across disciplines to develop and test models of complex interactions among biological, social, and behavioral processes in aging persons.

Interdisciplinary work also calls for databases that include both biological and psychosocial information. In addition to the empirical studies reported in this volume, there are a few other classic large scale epidemiological studies in differenct communities (e.g., Framingham, Tecumseh, Cleveland) that include a range of variables and could be used to add to our information about predictors of gender differences. Large scale epidemiological studies are useful for pointing to more in-depth examinations of the mechanisms linking biological, social, and behavioral factors to gender differences in morbidity and mortality.

These theoretical uncertainties and methodological limitations highlight the challenges in specifying the genetic, biological, social, and behavioral bases for the gender differential in health and longevity and predicting its future course. However, increased knowledge is important for understanding the causes and consequences of gender differences in longevity and for identifying ways of improving the health and functioning of both men and women.

The study of gender differences in health and longevity adds valuable information about the underlying social, behavioral, and biological bases for health and longevity. As such, gender studies should be viewed as a central area of research for understanding aging processes and the role of older people in society.

Index